FAST FACTS FOR THE CLINICAL NURSING INSTRUCTOR

Clinical Teaching in a Nutshell

D0104478

About the Authors

Eden Zabat Kan, DNSc, RN, received her bachelor's degree in nursing from the Penn State University at State College, PA, her master's degree in nursing education from Villanova University, Villanova, PA, and her doctorate in nursing science from Widener University, Chester, PA. She is currently employed in the ICCU at Civista Medical Center in LaPlata Maryland. Beginning Fall 2008, she will be teaching undergraduate students at the School of Nursing at The Catholic University of America in Washington DC. Prior to this position, she was a member of the faculty at West Chester University's Department of Nursing, where she coordinated clinical and didactic instruction for senior level undergraduate students. Her publications have been in the areas of medical surgical nursing, cardiac surgery, and nursing education.

Susan Stabler-Haas, MSN, RN, CS, LMFT, is an Assistant Professor of Nursing at West Chester University, PA, where she has been a faculty member since 1996. She is a graduate of Villanova University and has over twenty years of classroom and clinical teaching experience in the areas of medical-surgical, critical care, geriatric, and psychiatric nursing. Her instruction is influenced by her prior roles as staff nurse, rehab nurse, and critical care nurse manager in five Philadelphia area hospitals. She has educated students in a variety of nursing programs, including diploma, associate, baccalaureate, RN to BSN, and second degree nursing. Professor Stabler-Haas has also earned a Psychiatric Clinical Nurse Specialist designation from the University of Pennsylvania, and has been practicing as a licensed Marriage and Family Therapist.

FAST FACTS FOR THE CLINICAL NURSING INSTRUCTOR

Clinical Teaching in a Nutshell

Eden Zabat Kan, DNSc, RN
Susan Stabler-Haas, MSN, RN, CS, LMFT

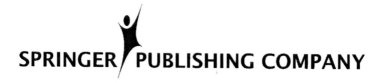

SPRINGER PUBLISHING COMPANY

New York

Springer Publishing Company, LLC
11 West 42nd Street
New York, NY 10036
www.springerpub.com

Acquisitions Editor: Allan Graubard
Production Editor: Barbara A. Chernow
Cover design: Joanne E. Honigman
Composition: Agnew's, Inc.

12/ 7

Library of Congress Cataloging-in-Publication Data

Kan, Eden Zabat.
    Fast facts for the clinical nursing instructor : clinical teaching in a nutshell / Eden Zabat Kan, Susan Stabler-Haas.
        p. ; cm.
    Includes bibliographical references and index.
    ISBN 978-0-8261-1887-5
    1. Nursing—Study and teaching. I. Stabler-Haas, Susan. II. Title.
    [DNLM: 1. Education, Nursing—methods. 2. Clinical Medicine. 3. Teaching—methods. WY 18 K1568s 2008]
    RT71.K28 2008
    610.73071'1—dc22

                        2008037752

Printed in the United States of America by IBT/Hamilton

Contents

Part III: Getting To Know Your Nursing Students: Who Are the Best, and Who Are the Rest?

Part IV: The Performance Appraisals: Clinical Evaluations

Part V: Communication at Clinical Conferences

Part VI: The Art of Making a Clinical Assignment

Part VII: Competencies Not Met

Foreword

Each of us has significant memories of our nursing school experience. Maybe we remember the clinical instructor who talked us through giving our first injection or inserting a Foley catheter. Maybe we remember "shaking in our boots" for fear that we would be unprepared to answer our instructor's questions. Maybe we remember the instructor we could approach with what we perceived to be a "stupid question." It is hoped that in all of these cases, we remember the importance of quality nursing and how much we learned from the instructors who dedicated their lives to providing positive learning experiences in the clinical setting. Although we might not be able to acknowledge these positive feelings as nursing students, we should come to appreciate the expertise of these faculty members in the clinical setting and remember our goal to achieve that same level of excellence.

The education of nursing students requires a balance between theoretical knowledge and clinical application—what some refer to as the science and art of nursing. Many nursing faculty members perform both of these roles within the nursing program, but as financial constraints increase, many colleges and universities have hired adjunct faculty who work only in the clinical facility with nursing students. Many of these individuals have significant clinical expertise, but they may lack the knowledge and skill to convey that expertise to students. Some faculty have not completed the graduate courses that support the teaching role, such as Curriculum, Tests and Measurements, Creative Teaching Strategies, and, most importantly, the Teaching Practicum experience, in which graduate students are placed in colleges and universities for a semester to learn the role of the nursing faculty member.

We all have to start somewhere, and I suspect some of you can remember your first clinical teaching position. The best clinical instructors make the job look easy, and most people don't realize how much effort goes into the process of clinical teaching that creates a positive learning environment for the nursing student. This book provides readers with a framework of ideas that will help them prepare for clinical teaching, including organizing the clinical experience, developing relationships with the staff in the clinical facilities, making clinical assignments, planning orientation days, developing clinical rotations, planning and facilitating pre- and postconferences, clinical evaluations, legal issues of clinical education and, of course, handling the student who is in jeopardy of failing the clinical course. The clinical instructor carries the additional burden of accountability—ensuring that each student is providing safe and effective nursing care to the patients. As a result, issues of personal liability and techniques for handling the student who is in jeopardy of giving unsafe care become important. Picture yourself teaching eight to ten nursing students on a busy medical surgical unit. If each student carries two to three patients, you quickly become aware of how challenging this responsibility can be. No wonder I have heard more than a few graduate students during their teaching practicum experience express surprise when they say, "I never knew how much work went into teaching!" I would be remiss if I didn't mention Teresa Christian as a shining example of these clinical nursing instructors. Many Villanova University alumni have described her as "tough, but the best instructor I ever had!"

The idea for this book began with discussions over coffee between two faculty members who had a similar philosophy about clinical instruction. They shared a commitment to making the clinical experience the best it could be for their students, making improvements each year they taught. In addition, they were often assigned the task of orienting and mentoring new clinical faculty. The authors agreed that what was missing in the literature was a "real-life" practical guide to assist new faculty in transitioning from clinical practice to clinical education. From those early discussions and a lot of brainstorming, this book became a reality.

This book serves as a valuable resource for nurses who are beginning their professional teaching careers and for seasoned faculty who seek additional resources to improve the clinical experience for their students. In many ways, this book is a tribute to the clinical aspects of our nursing programs and to the clinical faculty members who strive to make the student experience a positive one. This book was written by two of the best clinical faculty members I have ever known. I have learned much from them in my own practice, and I am confident that you will also grow from their combined experience and wisdom. There is no question that you will find among these pages a wealth of pragmatic, "real-life" information on the clinical teaching process.

I want to thank Susan Stabler Haas and Eden Zabat Kan for asking me to write the foreword for this book. It is indeed an honor to be a small part of this significant contribution to the nursing education literature. I am confident this book will help you to become one of those clinical instructors that students will look back on with pride and say, "That clinical instructor made me the nurse I am today!"

Susan C. Slaninka, EdD, RN
Adjunct Professor of Nursing
Villanova University College of Nursing

Preface

Let's face it. Not every nurse would make a good clinical instructor. Technical proficiency alone does not guarantee the ability to effectively manage nursing students at the clinical site. Even nurses who are capable of providing clinical instruction may not wish to take on the considerable personal liability associated with the oversight of these nursing students.

Perhaps you are different. Perhaps you are one of those nurses who is in fact both capable and willing to impart your knowledge to the next generation of caregivers. We commend you, for the future of our profession rests on your shoulders. After all, what is more important to the future of nursing than supervising and sharing our expertise with future nurses?

While personally rewarding, this vital role is also a formidable challenge. Clinical teaching is not easy. The expectations for an effective clinical nursing instructor are daunting. It can be a prodigious undertaking even for individuals with training or degrees in clinical instruction. They are continually faced with the changing demands of the patient and the challenges of adapting instruction to different learning styles. Moreover, most new clinical instructors do not have a solid foundation in teaching clinical courses. Indeed, many may not have any teaching experience. As a result, they face performance insecurities, along with the daily teaching challenges. It is easy to understand why nursing programs are pressed to fill their clinical instructor positions.

Our book, *Fast Facts for the Clinical Instructor: Clinical Teaching in a Nutshell,* represents thirty-two years of combined teaching experience. Designed as a practical guide for clinical instructors, it uses an "easy-to-follow" format. Each chapter provides information on key topics that should help ease the transition for the novice clinical nursing instructor, as well as provide alternate teaching approaches for the experienced instructor. Nuggets of pertinent information are summarized in boxes that present "Fast Facts in a Nutshell." The appendices provide valuable and useful material for the novice instructor. Instructors can preview templates that will assist them with organizing an orientation day, a clinical student assignment, and written assignments. In short, this book will help you, the clinical nursing instructor, introduce your students to their new career. It will provide guidance as you oversee their gradual development into professional caregivers. Finally, we hope that it provides the needed support and assistance you need to effectively teach future nurses in their clinical courses.

Eden Zabat Kan, DNSc, RN
Susan Stabler-Haas, MSN, RN, CS, LMFT

Acknowledgments

I am indebted to the many undergraduate and graduate students I have encountered over the years. You have all inspired me and are tied to my life forever. Thank you to all my friends and colleagues at West Chester University for giving me the support and friendship to become the teacher that I am today. Thank you for helping me make a living doing something that I love so much. I especially enjoyed working with Susan Slaninka. Thank you for taking my calls and sharing your wisdom when I needed it. You are proof that effective and successful teachers can also laugh and smile a lot. To my good friend Susan, it is still hard for me to believe that our many lunch or "after-clinical" chats about teaching in the clinical setting has led to this wonderful outcome. Thank you for being a true partner with this writing endeavor. I cherish our friendship. And finally to my wonderful husband, Dexter, I am blessed to have found you.

Eden Zabat Kan, DNSc, RN

I wish to thank all of my students whose feedback over the years has helped to shape this book. I also would like to thank my husband, Joe. Special thanks to Chris, my son, and my family and friends for all of their encouragement and support. To my coauthor, Eden, no one could ask for a better coauthor. Thanks to Susan Slaninka for all of her support over the years and for writing the Foreword to our book.

Susan Stabler-Haas, MSN, RN, CS, LMFT

Part I

Appreciating Your New Identity

From Caregiver to Educator

Chapter 1

Developing a New Identity as a Clinical Nursing Instructor

INTRODUCTION

Both the novice and the experienced nursing teacher need to modify their mindsets on many occasions. They need to shift their actions from the delivery of quality care of patients to the delivery of quality education to students who will one day provide patient care. This chapter introduces the "top ten" facts essential for clinical nursing instruction.

This chapter presents a questionnaire for your completion. After answering the questions, you will find explanatory information designed to enhance the development and refinement of your identity as a clinical nursing instructor.

In this chapter, you will learn:

1. How to begin the transition from staff nurse to clinical nursing instructor.
2. The basic facts of clinical teaching.

You have just begun a journey from staff nurse to clinical nursing instructor. Or, perhaps, you have been a nursing instructor who always felt the need for more information, more guidance, and more specific examples and plans to successfully instruct your students. Throughout this book, you will learn concrete and useful information that you can use immediately —even on the same day that you read it.

To begin, you should ask two questions:

1. What may be required for my transition from staff nurse to nursing clinical instructor?
2. Which of the following facts do I feel are important?

QUESTIONNAIRE

Place a T for true or an F for false next to the following facts below. Then, review the answers the that follow the questionnaire.

_____   1. I will need to prove my clinical competency on a daily basis.
_____   2. I will contribute to the nursing profession.
_____   3. I must be friends with my students.
_____   4. My students must always like me.
_____   5. The unit's staff nurses and aides should be happy to take guidance from me.
_____   6. I want to be familiar with the unit and the staff before I bring my students to the clinical setting.

_____ 7. I must know every detail about every client that my students care for.

_____ 8. I must supervise every procedure and almost all interactions between my students and patients.

_____ 9. I will earn much more money in this position.

_____ 10. All of my students will be motivated to learn as much as possible.

ANSWERS TO THE QUESTIONS: TRUE OR FALSE?

1. I will need to prove my clinical competency on a daily basis.

Some of you are transitioning from practice as expert staff nurses. Others are tenured professors, academic experts who need additional guidance in supervising students and in grasping the many facets of clinical instruction. Whatever your background, the first item for a clinical instructor to remember is that you will have to supervise clinical experiences with student nurses. The students you will encounter, whether in a two- or four-year program, are novice learners. Learning to refrain from performing any nursing skill or procedure for the student learner will be a major challenge. If the student is having a problem performing a basic clean dressing change on a wound, for example, you may be tempted to take over and complete the procedure. Resist taking over! Many seasoned clinical instructors will tell you, "Think more like a teacher and less like a nurse!" Your own professional goals of clinical competence should be tempered. Keep in mind that your role in the clinical setting is to enhance student learning by supervising (and not performing) skills. This involves using teaching learning strategies to enable the student to perform the clinical skill with knowledge and eventual competence.

An effective clinical instructor uses these strategies, such as "questioning," "role playing," and "interactive discussion," to improve students' thinking and problem solving skills. This is not an easy task. Being a good teacher requires much practice and learning.

Fast facts in a nutshell

- Think more like a teacher and less like a nurse!

---

2. I will contribute to the nursing profession.

Many nurses become clinical instructors without realizing that time is required to transition to the role. Part of the transition is learning the duties and values of that role. According to the AACN (2001), clinical instructors have, at a minimum, a practice focus and a commitment to decision making and critical thinking pedagogy. **The practice of clinical education is highly valued in this current environment of nursing shortages.** Whether you are a part-time or full time clinical instructor, you are contributing to a profession that is greatly in need of successful instructors who can teach students how to effectively care for their patients.

Fast facts in a nutshell

- The practice of clinical education is highly valued at this current environment of nursing shortages.

---

3. I must be friends with my students.

If you go into clinical teaching thinking that you can be "friends" with your students, then your tenure in this role will be short. As a result of the combined objective and subjective nature of clinical instruction and evaluation, friendships with your students can lead to difficult situations, particularly during the evaluation periods. Remember that each school's curriculum establishes many clinical objectives. If you share outside activities with students, you will expend energy that should be focused elsewhere—energy that should be used to enhance your students' clinical competence. In the unfortunate event that you may have to discipline or correct a student under your tutelage, it will be more difficult if you have not maintained the "boundary of teacher:student." **Keep personal information about yourself to a minimum.**

Fast facts in a nutshell

- Maintain the boundary of teacher:student.
- Keep personal information out of the clinical setting.

4. My students must always like me.

Face it, we all want to be liked as teachers. However, you should first focus on the clinical objectives for your students and place less emphasis on whether students "like" or even "appreciate" your efforts. Wouldn't you rather be the teacher who instills a memorable learning experience? **Focus instead on the "aha" moments of your students**—moments when your clinical thinking questions led to further student inquiry and successful application of concepts! Once you experience this moment, you will be hooked on teaching. You will realize that friendships and being "liked" cannot replace this feeling of accomplishment.

Fast facts in a nutshell

- Wait for the "aha" moments!

---

5. The unit's staff nurses and aides should be happy to take guidance from me.

Staff personnel, nurses, and aides are familiar with required routines at their clinical agencies and are knowledgeable about their work. Although they are not happy about changes in policy or procedures, they will adapt in time. Thus, they will eventually accept you and your students and be willing to alter their routines a bit. However, they will not be receptive to verbal direction or recommendations from a clinical instructor. If you want to communicate with the staff, ask the nurse manager for the proper procedure.

If, however, a staff member "corrects" you or a conflict develops, try to resolve the issue professionally. Although the staff nurses also model professional behavior, you are the daily role model for your students. Remember this when you observe a procedure that is being done incorrectly, and you want to provide input based on your practice experience. Recall that you are first a teacher and second a nurse. This is one of the hardest lessons to learn for beginning nurse instructors.

Your major goal as a clinical instructor is to teach your students. You are not there to teach the nurses or other ancillary staff! If you do so, your energy is being misdirected! Instead, direct all your energy to your students. You need some degree of humility. Your goal is to facilitate communication among staff and students, so steer clear of any conflicts. Rather, focus on teaching and preparing your students for success in the practice arena.

Fast facts in a nutshell

- You are not there to teach the nurses or other ancillary staff.

---

6. I want to be familiar with the unit and the staff before I bring my students to the clinical setting.

It is often a prudent practice to go for a "trial run" before you drive to an unfamiliar spot. For example, many people drive to the location of a job interview a day or two in advance to make sure that they know of any detours or potential problems on the route. Similarly, it is vital for any instructor, whether new to or familiar with the unit, to visit it before the first clinical orientation day with their students.

Call the nurse manager and arrange to come for at least half a day. He/she may meet with you for a brief period, during which you should be prepared to explain the clinical objectives of the course and provide the names of the students with clinical hours. Also be prepared to ask questions. It is her/his "turf!" You are a guest! Remember that!

You may want to go through a "full shift" with a willing, veteran nurse, thereby becoming "familiar with the culture" and routines of the unit. The bonus is clear: You will have an experienced nurse ally waiting for you when you return with your students.

Fast facts in a nutshell

- Become familiar with the unit and the staff before the arrival of your students.

---

7. I must know every detail about every client that my students care for.

No, you do not! Remember that the staff nurse is ultimately responsible for the patients. Not you! You need to know times of medications, safety information like "code status," NPO status, necessary lab specimens, general diagnoses, and precautions, such as isolation standards. You cannot know all there is to know about the ten plus patients, with at least seven to eight students in your group.

Encourage your students to assume the responsibility for learning about their patients. It is the student who needs to feel the "pressure" of the obligation to thoroughly read the nursing documentation forms and check with the primary nurse about the patient. Your job is to foster and encourage the students to gather the information and remember it throughout their clinical day.

Fast facts in a nutshell

- Encourage students to be responsible by thoroughly reading each patient's chart, medication list, and careplan.

---

8. I must supervise every procedure and almost all interactions between my students and patients.

You would be setting yourself up for failure and frustration very quickly if you try to practice this philosophy. While you will need to supervise most medication administration, intravenous medication responsibilities, new procedures (e.g., insertion of a urinary Foley catheter, insertion of a nasogastric tube, changing of a sterile dressing), you cannot be everywhere all of the time.

In fact, depending on your schedule, you may sometimes allow the staff nurse to supervise your student in putting in a urinary Foley catheter or changing a sterile dressing. For example, you may be supervising one student's administration of intravenous medications when you are notified that another student needs to place a urinary catheter into her patient immediately. If you have established a rapport with the primary nurse whom you believe to be trustworthy and professional and he/she offers to supervise your student, allow it to happen. **You need to trust your staff nurses** while broadening your students' experiences.

Fast facts in a nutshell

- You cannot be everywhere all of the time.

---

9. I will be making much more money in this position.

Wrong! You may very likely earn less money initially than your graduating seniors do. This is not a lucrative field, except in the area of satisfaction. As we mentioned earlier, when one of your students gets that "aha" moment, it will be worth the pay cut. Remember also that you will be working an academic year, which is only eight months a year in most settings. You will have opportunities to teach in the summer and develop new courses, which can boost your financial and self-esteem accounts. If you choose to enter the tenured track in an academic institution, your salary will increase incrementally and also more quickly. If you work in an academic institution that has union representation for its professors, this is more likely to be true.

Many opportunities exist to increase your income. You can publish, work as a staff nurse during periods off, consult and work part time for one clinical rotation in a different nursing school. All of these expand your horizons. This is an important judgment call for you.

Fast facts in a nutshell

- Financial gain should not motivate you to become a clinical instructor. Rather, your motive should be to skillfully and effectively teach students to be successful nurses.

---

10. All of my students will be motivated to learn as much as possible.

Sad to say, this is not always the case. Some students will have other life issues that interfere with their ability to devote the time and energy needed to a clinical nursing rotation. Others may not have realized what "nursing" really encompasses and may stay in the major just to graduate and get a job. These students, however, will be in the minority. You will receive satisfaction from the wonderful students who truly are motivated to learn and will work extremely hard under your guidance. They are the future nurses of whom you will be proud and who will make teaching worthwhile for you. **There is no greater satisfaction than to realize that your former students are surpassing you in knowledge**—that they have become nurses whom you would want to care for you and for your family.

Fast facts in a nutshell

- You are helping to educate nurses whom you would want to care for you and your family.

Chapter 2

Understand the Rules:
What Every Nursing Instructor Needs to Know about the Nursing Program's Policies

INTRODUCTION

This chapter discusses the importance of the academic policies at your clinical setting and the specific information that will prove useful to the clinical instructor. The discussion emphasizes that the clinical instructor is responsible for enforcing these policies among his or her students. The chapter begins with a true/false exercise that will enable you to review your baseline knowledge about clinical instruction.

In this chapter, you will learn:

1. The clinical instructor tasks that must be completed before starting the clinical practicum with students.
2. What information is key to the success of the clinical instructor.

KNOW YOUR BASELINE

Start by answering the true/false questions in Exhibit 2.1. Remember that all **clinical instructors must complete a comprehensive examination of their school's nursing program** before actually starting the clinical days with students. By the time the instructor is hired, the dean or the nursing program

---

EXHIBIT 2.1   True/False Exercise

For each statement below, check either true or false.

True   False

True	False	
____	____	1. Clinical teaching involves no advance preparation.
____	____	2. Familiarity with the nursing program is a priority before your first clinical day with students.
____	____	3. The student handbook is one of the most important resources for all clinical instructors.
____	____	4. Policies of academic work are not usually found in the student handbook.
____	____	5. At the time of hire, you should not expect to receive any written materials about the nursing program.

Answers to True/False questions: 1. False; 2. True; 3. True; 4. False; 5. False

chairperson will probably have supplied a clinical packet containing essential materials, such as a description of job responsibilities, the faculty handbook, the student handbook, and the course catalog. The instructor is expected to study these materials and return with any questions. It is normal hire etiquette to provide new clinical faculty with the following:

Essential Clinical Materials
  A. Clinical Packet
         Clinical course syllabus
         Clinical Practicum or Academic Calendar Schedule
         Clinical Assignment Sheet
         Clinical Evaluation Tool (Student and Professor)
         Diagnostic Medication and Calculation Quiz
         (a sample copy)
  B. Faculty Handbook/Manual
         Clinical Job Responsibilities highlighted
  C. Student Handbook - Clinical Policies
         Grading Policy
         Dress Code Policy
         Attendance Policy
         Tardiness Policy
         Safe/Unsafe Practice Policy

THE CLINICAL PACKET

The clinical packet is usually a folder of sheets or forms that may include the current course syllabus, an academic calendar or dates of the practicum, and, if possible, certain helpful forms, such as a blank clinical assignment sheet or a copy of a medication quiz (for an example, go to www.alysion.org/dimensional/analysis.htm#problems). This packet also often contains the clinical evaluation tool that will be used to grade each student. As this tool is generally filed in the student's folder at the conclusion of the practicum, be sure you understand how to use it. For an example of a clinical packet, go to www.dixie.edu/health/nursing/pdfsyllab/1105.pdf.

If you receive the student handbook and faculty manual, but not a clinical packet, contact the person who hired you. In some programs, this information is available electronically on the nursing program's Web site. Your program dean or chairperson should refer you to someone who can assist in obtaining necessary information. At some nursing schools, instructors may also be assigned a contact person, who is usually a full-time senior faculty member with relevant experience in the clinical practicum. This contact person can provide the clinical packet of information, assist you in interpreting the clinical evaluation tool, and inform you of any new program updates or changes. The clinical instructor is usually a "clinical only" faculty member, which means that the job may not require attendance at faculty meetings or certain school functions. In some programs, the information is relayed electronically through e-mail. It is the duty of the clinical instructor to keep himself or herself informed about the student functions of the nursing program.

COURSE CATALOG

Furthermore, you may also receive the course catalog. Most course catalogs are now available for public access online; many are printed annually or every two years. The catalog contains courses and programs, as well as the academic requirements for each program. For example, an undergraduate course catalog will list all the courses offered in each undergraduate program, including nursing, along with a brief description of each course.

STUDENT HANDBOOK

Of all the resources the clinical instructor receives, **the student handbook is probably the most valuable and important.** In most programs, a student handbook is developed by the faculty in cooperation with students in that nursing program. It is an outstanding resource for all clinical instructors primarily because it spells out the policies and procedures relating to academic student work. In addition, the handbook contains information about the nursing program and curriculum. It describes not only the program's policies, but also its mission, philosophy, and main goals, as required by accrediting bodies. All nursing schools require accreditation.

Program Goals

Clinical instructors are encouraged to understand their school's goals for its students. There may be times when you are asked to share information about your school with others. For example, patients or hospital staff may be curious about the school's general program and policies. However, the most important reason to carefully examine the handbook is that it contains explicit instructions for the clinical aspects of the program.

Dress and Attendance Policies

Most health care agencies have policies on everything from dress codes to continuing attendance education. **Familiarize yourself with the school's policies because you will be required to enforce them at the clinical site.** One that you will need to enforce every day is the dress code! Students must adhere to this dress code, which is usually carefully monitored and evaluated. This code may specify dress attire, jewelry limitations, hair and nail length, facial piercing, hair color, and other aspects of one's appearance. Adherence to the dress code is identified in a student's clinical evaluation under objectives that specify "professional behavior."

The student handbook also identifies policies on absences, tardiness, and clinical practice expectations. There is usually a zero tolerance for absences or tardiness. Each and every clinical day is considered vital to the overall program. Lateness for the clinical day is always frowned upon. Tardiness and absences are further discussed in Chapter 16.

Program Expectations

Of course, some programs provide more and some provide less information in their student handbooks. Another item that you may find is the clinical practice expectations for each level of the program. In a four-year nursing program, for example, basic expectations for the second-year student will be different from those for the third-year or senior student. In addition, each clinical site has setting-specific rules and policies. That is, the policies and procedures for a medical surgical setting will be different from those in the community health clinical rotation. Students will usually receive this information from their clinical instructor at orientation or on their first day at the facility. Chapter 4 provides an outline on the necessary and general information that must be shared with students on orientation day.

Yes, most clinical instructors agree that **the student handbook is the first item to be reviewed, as it is usually considered the "bible."** The novice instructor will probably focus initially on his or her job responsibilities, but the expert will quickly find and read the handbook. To begin the clinical rotation with students and start planning learning experiences and activities for them, the instructor needs a basic understanding of the school and its student policies. The student handbook is a solid starting place for that information. In addition, the majority of student handbooks are now posted online for public review. For example, refer to that from the University of Illinois at Chicago School of Nursing <http://www.uic.edu/nursing/oap/stumanual/index.htm>.

CLINICAL PRACTICUM

Exhibit 2.2 is an example of a checklist that may help guide what must be done before the first day of the clinical practicum.

EXHIBIT 2.2   Instructor's Checklist

To Do . . .
Instructor's Checklist

_____ Understand Job Responsibilities
_____ Familiarize yourself with the Student Handbook
        Understand the Mission and Philosophy
        Read the basic policies and procedures
_____ Visit the Agency
        Meet with the Nurse Manager
        Tour the Unit
        Meet with the Staff Personnel
_____ Obtain access
        Computers for Lab Values
        Medication Systems (Pyxis)
        Electronic Documentation Systems

Fast facts in a nutshell

- Before the clinical practicum begins, make contact with your faculty resource.
- Understand the nursing program's goals and curriculum as highlighted in the student handbook.
- Before orientation day with students, have a clear understanding of the student policies applicable to your clinical course.

Part II

Your Success Depends on "Y O U" Preparing for Your Clinical Teaching Assignment

Chapter 3

You Are a Guest, So Act like One

INTRODUCTION

Your success depends on "YOU!" This is the first chapter to discuss the essential and "lifesaving" relationship between the clinical instructor and the clinical unit staff. The unit to which you are assigned is NOT a classroom. It is the nursing staff's turf. You are a guest. This chapter provides two examples of novice instructors with different techniques in the clinical setting. You decide whose approach is the most effective and, therefore, which you would adopt.

In this chapter, you will learn:

1. The art of recognizing the expertise of each nurse and how to approach each nurse as an expert (even if you disagree with something).
2. Information that can "make or break" a clinical instructor.
3. How to effectively interact with the nursing staff.

YOU ARE A GUEST, SO ACT LIKE ONE

The clinical site is not an alternative classroom nor should it be considered the teacher's turf. The clinical site is a nursing unit (or agency) and, therefore, the domain of the nurses who staff it. Your role as clinical instructor does not alter the fact that you are ultimately a guest on their floor. Your goal is to establish the essential and professional "lifesaving" relationship between you and the unit's nursing staff.

The patients whom the students will care for are the responsibility of the unit's staff nurses and technicians. Accede to their sovereignty over patient care. Although rarely discussed in graduate school, this largely unspoken rule is integral to the success of the clinical nursing instructor. **Always acknowledge the staff nurses as the experts in rendering care to their patients,** even if circumstances may occasionally cause you to question that expertise. The importance of adopting the proper approach in relating to the nursing staff is illustrated in Exhibits 3.1 and 3.2, which offer two examples of nursing instructors who are about to bring their students into a new unit.

CASE STUDIES: INTRODUCING STUDENTS TO THE CLINICAL SETTING AND STAFF

EXHIBIT 3.1   Bob's Approach

Bob is a new hire, eager to begin his first position as a clinical nursing instructor. He has been a critical care nurse for the last two years and recently completed his master's degree. He is also new to the facility to which he will bring his first group of students and has called the nurse manager to arrange a meeting with her. He tells the manager that the students will take only patients who are oriented to person, place, and time, and who are able to communicate clearly. He also informs the manager that the students will NOT be helping the clients with their morning care or with any hygiene needs. Bob states, "The students are here to learn their future professional role and that does not include bed-making and baths." The manager terminates the meeting abruptly and tells Bob that she thinks there may be a conflict with accommodating his students since a different school of nursing may also be scheduled for the same days. Bob is almost apoplectic, stammering that his students should have priority. The meeting ends badly.

EXHIBIT 3.2   Mary's Approach

Mary has five years of experience as a home health nurse and has two more courses to complete for her master's degree. She has gathered information about the home health agency to which she will soon be bringing her students and has arranged to meet with the nurse manager. Mary's students will be working with the agency's nurses and going on home visits with them. Mary explains the objectives of the nursing course to the nurse manager. She details her own experience and acquaints him with the level of expertise of her new students. She requests that the manager tell her which nurses would be most appropriate for the students to accompany on their home care visits. She stresses that the students are prepared to perform many functions under the direct supervision of the professional nurses with whom they are paired. Mary uses the meeting as an opportunity to compliment the nurse manager for allowing students to have this learning experience. Finally, Mary offers to join a nurse herself for one or two visits before the students begin their rotation, so that mutual expectations might be realistically set. The manager arranges for Mary to spend a half-day with one of her more experienced nurses and also states that he will discuss the students' impending arrival at the next agency staff meeting. When he meets with his staff, he intends to highlight the mutual benefits of this professional/student interaction and promises to call back with the names of the nurses who will mentor these students.

Lessons Learned from the Case Studies

Based on these case studies, answer the following questions:

- Which nursing instructor will be successful?
- Which technique received the most positive reaction and feedback?
- Which students will have the best learning experience?

Unlike Bob, **Mary clearly understood that she was a "guest" at the clinical site.** She inquired about the agency and apprised the manager about the students' abilities. She asked the manager to assign nurses who really wanted to work with students, thus allowing the staff nurses to have input into the mentoring process. If the members of the nursing staff are given a choice and a voice in teaching (or not teaching) students, it will result in a better experience for the students—and the instructor.

Fast facts in a nutshell

- You are a guest; act like one.
- Positive relationships with the nursing staff are paramount.
- Staff nurses are ultimately responsible for the patients.

Chapter 4

Organize the Semester – Have a Plan

INTRODUCTION

An instructor is required to review the rules and requirements of the facility where they conduct each clinical rotation. The goal of the chapter is to provide blueprints for the first day of a clinical rotation. Each rotation can last from four days to seven weeks, meeting twice a week.

As each instructor spends most of the first day preparing written expectations and guidelines for students, this chapter presents a template of an orientation day schedule. The sample guides and rules are adaptable to any setting. They have been developed by the authors and used by them quite effectively.

In this chapter, you will learn:

1. How to organize and conduct your first day with your clinical students.
2. Which blueprints can be most effectively used with the written guidelines to enhance your students' orientation to the unit and an understanding of their responsibilities.

FIRST DAY OF THE SEMESTER

After your own orientation to the new unit, you can begin to develop your plan for the first day on the floor with your students. Think ahead! You must **find a way to communicate to your students** when and where you will meet on their first day. After all, the educational experience can be greatly diminished if they don't show up! Here are some possibilities for getting the word out:

- Ask the level coordinator to announce the time and place of the first meeting to your group at the facility, as well as to provide maps and directions online.
- Meet the group members at the school when they have class and provide the same information.
- Use the school's e-mail to provide the initial information.

The goal is to **ensure that your clinical group clearly understands the place, time, and attire for the first clinical day.** Be clear. Instead of saying, "meet me in the lobby of the building," be specific. Say, instead, "meet me in front of the big clock in the Smith lobby at 8 AM sharp!" Provide a map with written directions. Don't forget about nourishment. Often this is a four- to six-hour day, so inform them about the lunch possibilities or dinner if you are supervising an evening clinical. Look at Appendix A for further guidelines to assist you on orientation day.

ORGANIZE

Reserving Space

You must reserve space at the clinical site to conduct your orientation. Most hospitals have a limited number of conference rooms, so you may need to speak with the level coordinator. However, it is more likely that you, the clinical instructor, will have to obtain that information yourself, either from the nurse educator or the manager assigned to your clinical site.

Whether you will be instructing for eight days or eight weeks, **an ORGANIZED and thorough orientation day will reap dividends** throughout the semester and promote a successful and enjoyable clinical experience for you, your students, and the patients and staff with whom you will be working.

Orientation Day

The first time your clinical group meets should be an orientation day, an evaluation-free period during which **instructors show their students the clinical site and clearly explain performance expectations.** Students will naturally be anxious on their first few days at your site. If you take a day or a few hours to review the clinical course and show students where to find certain equipment, their anxieties will ease. Consider using the orientation template that appears on the next few pages. It has been refined and polished over our thirty plus years of clinical instruction. It is adaptable to any setting and any type of nursing program.

ORIENTATION DAY TEMPLATE

A. Begin with an Icebreaker

Students often know each other only superficially, if at all. **This makes team-building an essential first step.** Your team members must work cohesively if they are to learn the maximum in their short time with you. One example of an icebreaker would be to ask each student to write down on a card two things that the group does not know about him or her. Have each student (including you) choose a card and try to guess which student the card belongs to. You, as the instructor, should also participate in this activity. This will enhance your relationship with your students and help the group members become more comfortable with one another.

B. Ask each student to define his or her goals for the clinical practicum rotation

Collect this information from your students. Give each student a copy of their response, and keep one for yourself. If you have this information early in the day, you can better gauge and redefine student expectations. The level coordinator may have given you objectives and goals, but the students may have completely different ideas. If such a discrepancy exists, you need to adjust your orientation by better educating students about the school and the coordinator's objectives. Flexibility is paramount in this role.

C. Confirm their mathematical competency

If students are administering medications in the clinical practicum, it is prudent to give them a brief and simple medication calculation quiz that requires knowledge of basic math, such as ratio and proportion and intravenous drip rate equations. Students should be reminded that almost **every new registered nurse in a healthcare facility must pass a medication calculation** quiz as a condition of hire. Be sure to acquaint them with the basic abbreviations used by the institution for the protection of you and the patients. For example, Q.I.D. means 4 times a day, but you should specify what four times your institution designates as appropriate, for example, 8, 12, 1600, 2000. This cursory evaluation allows you to see if some students need to be sent back to the learning lab for review before they are allowed to administer medications.

D. Establish the course requirements

Like students everywhere, your charges want to know the "bottom line." What do we have to do to pass this clinical rotation? It is a key question, and you should not hesitate to address it. Each clinical instructor brings his or her personality and style to the instruction. **The students need to know what you judge important for their success.** Clinical rotations may be pass/fail or result in an letter or numeric grade. All students need a copy of the school's clinical evaluation tool at the outset of the clinical experience, and you should review each line or item with them. Part IV reviews the types of grading systems.

E. Key components

The following **key components** must be included in your verbal presentation and in any handouts to students.

- The clinical hours that are required, for example, Tuesdays and Thursdays from 7 AM to 1 PM.
- The required dates of the clinical rotation. Include any school events or holidays on which there no clinical days.
- The essential expectations that you and the nursing program manager deem most important. For example, attendance and punctuality may be the most basic criteria for assessing performance. If students are not present or not on time, it is difficult to assess performance. Remind them this is all part of their professionalism.
- Contact information should be provided. If the student will be late or absent, how and when do you require them to notify you and the unit? If they need to contact you at other times during the week, tell them the best way, such as e-mail or phone.
- Give sample documentation flow sheets to the students. These are the forms your students will use to write their assessments and notes. If your institution uses electronic charting, first familiarize yourself with this system and then adapt it to your students' needs. Find out if each student can receive a password to gain entry into the documentation system. The students will need practice with this skill.
- Journals may also be required. See Appendix B for an instructor's template of written journal requirements.

F. Emphasize the students' responsibilities while in the unit

The nurses in your unit must be confident that your students will properly discharge all their responsibilities before you all leave the unit. For example, if you agree to have the students document a full assessment, perform hygiene care, and administer medication, you must ensure that these tasks are completed before you and the students end the day. If it is not, the staff will become distrustful and disinclined to allow you or your students to care for their patients. They may also hesitate to teach and share knowledge with you students. One fact cannot be overemphasized—**the instructor's relationship with the staff and nurse unit manager is paramount for a successful clinical experience** for the students and for the instructor. Post a written guide to the staff of the student's responsibilities while on the unit.

G. Take the tour

At the beginning or end of orientation day, the instructor may schedule a visit to the unit. If you arrange this visit at the end of the day, remember that students may have already reached their saturation point for absorbing information. You may only be able to give them a handout with essential codes to use to gain entry into kitchens, utility rooms, and med rooms. The handout can include a sample schedule of their clinical day or a list of their patients (see Appendix C for a sample student schedule). Another suggestion is to let the students review a patient chart and have them walk around and tour the unit on their own.

Fast facts in a nutshell

- Be organized and have a plan for orientation day.
- Provide detailed written information, and distribute a copy to students.
- Ensure that all student responsibilities are completed before leaving the unit each day.

Chapter 5

Confidentiality and Patient Privacy

INTRODUCTION

Use discretion always. In other words, do not talk about patients in the elevators, in public spaces, or in front of individuals not specifically designated by the patient to receive information.

This chapter provides, specific examples of students who violated patient privacy by speaking "innocently" about their patients outside of the clinical setting. Information will be given about maintaining patient privacy while delivering care in the unit.

In this chapter, you will learn:

1. Relevant provisions of the Health Insurance Portability and Accountability Act (HIPAA) and how it interfaces with your students.
2. Ways in which students can violate patient privacy.
3. Basic suggestions to avoid violations of privacy.

CONCEPTS OF CONFIDENTIALITY
AND PATIENT PRIVACY

The concept of confidentiality in health care enjoys widespread acceptance in the United States (Potter & Perry, 2005). **Maintaining the confidentiality of client healthcare information is both a legislative and professional imperative**, as underscored by the Health Insurance Portability and Accountability Act of 1996 (HIPAA) and the American Nurses Association Code of Ethics. HIPAA was designed to increase the confidentiality of patient information.

Students may be on the same units as their neighbors, peers, or family and friends. It cannot be emphasized enough that absolutely NO information about any client/patient can be discussed with anyone outside of the unit's perimeter. When a breach occurs, litigation can follow.

Teaching the Concepts

Most nursing programs teach the concepts of patient privacy and confidentiality in the classroom. Your students may be aware of HIPAA and patient privacy, but the practice of privacy in the clinical field is another matter. As a nursing instructor, you must educate your students and monitor their discussions to ensure that the privacy of each client is protected. Never hesitate to impress on your new charges how vital patient privacy truly has become.

The **goal is to apply the theory taught on HIPAA to the clinical field.** That is, the clinical instructor must ascertain the degree of student understanding and, most importantly, how HIPAA laws apply to the clinical setting. In an acute care setting, for example, there are multiple times when a student may encounter visitors at their patient's bedsides. They have to be careful to whom they speak and what information they convey to these visitors. There have been occasions on which visiting family and neighbors received health information that they should not have been given.

Case Studies

Case Studies 5.1 and 5.2 present two different scenarios that emphasize the need for each instructor to stress daily to students that **client confidentiality is paramount**.

As these cases demonstrate, the aphorism that encourages the "ounce of prevention" rings especially true in the clinical setting. One must also emphasize the need for privacy while on the unit itself. This means that all computer screens must be turned off when students are not using them. If a visitor simply walks past an unattended screen and inadvertently sees a patient name and information, a violation of privacy has occurred and liability could possibly result for those at the nursing station.

CASE STUDY 5.1   Hannah's Scenario

During Hannah's geriatric rotation, she cared for an eighty-year-old patient. She did an excellent job and was complimented by her instructor and by the staff. She went home and told her family how

(continued)

much she enjoyed caring for her client and what happened during her day. She mentioned the patient's name to her family, thinking that he lived in a different town and that no one could possibly know him. Based on the circumstances of the patient's case, the student's mother correctly concluded that the patient was in fact the father of one of her employees. This worker had missed a lot of time lately supposedly because of personal illness. She became angry that her employee was not ill as she had claimed, but rather was taking time off to be with her father. The student was very concerned that her mother would reprimand the staff member, causing the employee to subsequently question how the mother had obtained this information. The student now wondered if she needed to inform her nursing instructor of the confidentiality breach.

CASE STUDY 5.2   Grace's Scenario

Grace had to present her client to her clinical group and was preparing the presentation in her dormitory room. She had her patient's name on all of the information that she was preparing and left the presentation material on her desk. Later in the day, her former high school friends came to visit and planned to stay overnight in her room. One friend read the information on her desk and exclaimed that the patient was her boyfriend's mother. She also said that her boyfriend does not live with his mother and was not aware of his mother's clinical psychiatric situation. She began to call him on her cell phone to inform him that his mom was in a psychiatric facility. Grace pleaded with her to not call and tried to explain how she would be in serious trouble if this information about the client was revealed.

Family Members

Another potential problem involves the information that you can share with family members of the patient. It is the patient —not the provider—who controls the disclosure of information to any individual not involved in his or her care. You must **procure the patient's permission before you can discuss his or her medical condition with the family.** If family members are present in the room and the client asks you questions, you are still on somewhat shaky ground. It is prudent to discuss with clients beforehand what information they want discussed and shared with family members. If you have any doubts, ask the family to briefly leave the room and then ask the client to clarify what areas are acceptable to discuss. You can also ask the client to sign a consent form before the discussion takes place, especially if sensitive material is to be discussed. Information about acquired immunodeficiency syndrome, sexually transmitted diseases, substance abuse, and psychiatric illness are considered especially sensitive.

Fast facts in a nutshell

- Always use discretion concerning client privacy.
- No information should be divulged without consent.
- Before sharing information with families, confer with patients.

Part III

Getting To Know
Your Nursing Students

Who Are the Best and
Who Are the Rest?

Chapter 6

The High Fliers:
How to Screen for
Higher Achieving Students

INTRODUCTION

One of the challenging aspects of clinical teaching is managing students during the limited blocks of time available for instructor observation. Practicing nurses work 8 or 12 hour shifts, whereas, student nurses are usually at the clinical sites for 4 to 8 hour blocks of time. As a result, many clinical instructors try to see things "early." That is, most seasoned clinical instructors try to identify or classify their students within the first week of the clinical rotation. One such classification would be students "at risk" (at risk for failing the course) and students "not at risk."

In this chapter you will learn:

1. The characteristics of students who are not at risk, those who are considered "high fliers."
2. The advantages of classifying students early in the program.

ASSESSING STUDENT CAPABILITIES

The clinical instructor is first and foremost a teacher. To become an effective teacher, the instructor must assist students to learn to problem solve and think at a higher level. Therefore, the successful instructor needs to develop quick insight into the nature and capabilities of the students. Within the first two weeks of the clinical rotation, the instructor should be able to distinguish between the higher fliers, those who will potentially receive higher grades, and the not-so-high fliers, or at risk students, who are in the bottom half of the group.

IDENTIFYING THE HIGH FLIERS

This distinction is also important because the clinical instructor faces certain stresses when dealing with a student who is at risk for failing the clinical course. The first sign of possible failure is unsatisfactory behavior when performing a nursing skill. The instructor needs to take extra time to manage this behavior while continuing to teach the other students within the time frame set by the nursing program.

Surprisingly, for some instructors, identifying the high fliers is quite easy. Some use instinct. For example, some students may impress you by completing homework earlier than the rest of the group or by earning a high grade on the medication quiz. Sometimes, a student's question may give you an impression of that student's cognitive ability. For example, one student may ask, "I just took vitals on my patient. What do I do next? In comparison, another student may voice, "I took vitals on my patient. Now I am starting the nursing assessment because I plan to give the medications soon." Obviously, the second student has a clear understanding of the nursing process and can initiate interventions competently. Initiating interventions competently is a major objective for student nurses, as it is a basic requirement and goal of graduation. This goal, as well as other goals for students, is usually documented in the student handbook of most nursing programs.

CHARACTERISTICS OF HIGH FLIERS

Based on years of experience and bearing witness to all kinds of student behaviors, the following are the most **common characteristics of "high fliers."**

1. The **student is prepared** each clinical day and displays this during the clinical rotation.

This student has reviewed his or her patient assignment and has some knowledge base to share with you about the patient's condition. If assigned to give medications that day, he or she will have medications reviewed and written down. This student may even present you with pages of written or typed notes of the work he or she did in preparing for the clinical day. Those papers will include information about the patient's medical disease process and the management of the medications. Each medication the patient is prescribed may be documented. The student will also bring his or her own books to the clinical facility.

2. The **student communicates** well orally with you and the patients.

This student asks you questions about the patient and can clearly verbalize some information about the assigned patient. When observed, this student is comfortable at the bedside speaking to the patient and the staff nurses. The student may show initiative by, for example, using the Internet to research such topics as smoking cessation or dietary needs, such as foods that are high in fiber.

3. The **student prioritizes patient interventions appropriately**.

For example, in a medical surgical dayshift rotation, without your direction, you witness the student rechecking a heart rate because the patient complained of dizziness. Another example is at a community rotation, where the student may check the vital signs and promptly report to you or the staff nurse an abnormal blood pressure and heart rate. This student may even ask a staff nurse to recheck the vital signs with him or her for accuracy.

Fast facts in a nutshell

- Clinical instructors can become effective teachers.
- It is best to distinguish the high fliers early.
- High fliers are prepared, communicate at a higher level, and can prioritize nursing interventions better.

Chapter 7

The Not-So-High Fliers:
How to Screen for Potential
"Problem Students"

INTRODUCTION

Teaching in the clinical setting requires an enormous amount of preparation before the course begins and then prior to each clinical day. One major frustration for instructors is the limited time available at the clinical site to teach all the students. In some acute care settings, the instructor to student ration is a surprising ten to one. State Boards of Nursing are well aware of this fact. One practice that can assist the clinical instructor is the "early identification" of strong students (high fliers) and weak students (not so high fliers).

In this chapter, you will learn:

1. The characteristics of the not-so high fliers.
2. How to compare high fliers and "not-so-high fliers."

IDENTIFYING "AT-RISK" STUDENTS

Instructors need to "see it early" according to Teeter (2001). That is, they need to **identify the at-risk students or the not-so-high fliers by certain "red flags."** Some of these red flags are: "The student arrives late on the first or second day," or the student is "unengaged with learning" or the student "frequently gets staff and other students to help" (p. 91). Sometimes, you may at first think that some students have really good relationships with the staff of nurses, nurse assistants, and technicians, particularly as you witness their close interactions. But this can be a warning sign. It is wise to keep an extra eye on these students just to make sure that they are doing their work and not just "copying" data from what has already been documented. They could even be getting answers (to your questions) from the staff nurses!

"Seeing it early" is a good strategy to employ as a clinical instructor. The not-so-high fliers may be more difficult to notice. Develop a keen sense of awareness. For example, some instructors might automatically stigmatize students who stay at the patient's bedside or are difficult to find during the clinical day. However, these students may not be at risk. Yes it's true that students who are nowhere to be found may be "hiding" from you and your questions about their care, but that student may also just be spending their time caring for their assigned patient and being extremely attentive to the needs of that patient. You need to discern these differences.

CHARACTERISTICS OF "NOT-SO-HIGH FLIERS"

Here are a few characteristics of the not-so-high fliers and a discussion of each, which are listed in Table 7.1.

1. The **student is not thoroughly prepared** each clinical day.

In most cases, there is a great deal of self-directed preparation on behalf of the student. Not-so-high fliers, however, will be unprepared even though they may have been instructed to prepare for a particular procedure, such as foley catheter insertion or medication shot. Another example is assigned written work. Whatever the case, the not-so-high fliers will not turn in their work or will turn in work that is incomplete.

TABLE 7.1 High Fliers vs. Not-so-High-Fliers	
High Fliers	Not-So-High-Fliers
1. Prepared for each clinical day	1. Not thoroughly prepared for the clinical day.
2. Communicates clearly with instructor and/or patients and staff nurses	2. Inconsistent with communication (for example, may not have verbalized to you an abnormal vital sign)
3. Prioritizes patient interventions appropriately	3. Unsure about patient care priorities.

Whether the assignment is written or oral, the not-so-high fliers will have an excuse as to why their performance is not up to par and why they are "unprepared." More likely than not, the clinical instructor will witness such a student sitting in the back of a nursing lounge with an open textbook, writing down the information that he or she should have arrived with at beginning of the clinical day.

2. The **student is inconsistent in communicating** information (for example, the student may not have informed you of a patient with a high BP value).

The not so high fliers are less assertive than the others in the group. That is, they are more comfortable being spoken to than actually initiating a conversation with you! As a result, they may not convey information promptly. They may know they are hearing something abnormal in the lungs or note a higher BP value in a patient, but they cannot decide what the next step should be. They do not speak to the staff nurse or a fellow student to seek their feedback. In fact, instead of speaking to anyone about their suspicions, they keep the information to themselves.

The instructor should note that what may be alarming about this characteristic is that inadequate communication may be the result of inherent shyness and not a lack of knowledge or preparation. Therefore, the instructor must do some careful probing before judging the student's potential. Although students who are shy do not have the same eye contact or nonverbal behavior than the others, this does not always mean they are not-so-high fliers. Further questioning of the student in a private place or at your office may be warranted to gain a bit more understanding of the student. Taking away part of the anxiety (being in the role of a clinical student during a clinical performance day) may actually help you to get more insight into your student.

3. The student is unsure about patient care priorities.

Every clinical rotation has expectations of basic student competencies and skills. It is expected that students advance through each rotation and make improvements within a given clinical rotation. This is most true in medical surgical settings where nurses care for multiple patients with various medical needs. Nurses are taught to prioritize their actions. They learn this skill during clinical rotations with clinical instructors.

The not-so-high fliers struggle with prioritizing basic care for their patients. To them, every intervention is a priority. A morning bath may be more important than getting the morning vital signs. Providing the evening snack as soon as it arrives may be more important then checking if the patient is diabetic and needs insulin first. They may not know that assessment of heart sounds is a priority action before administering a prescribed beta blocker medication. This problem with prioritization may either be a thinking problem or a problem related to self-induced anxiety. For example, a patient may have just woken up and asked the student to set up a bath. Not thinking through the care tasks for the day, the student happily helps the patient get this done before all other assessments.

MONITOR "NOT-SO-HIGH FLIERS"

Once you have some idea of which student or students are the "not-so-high fliers" in your clinical group, keep a critical eye on them. That's it! It is also wise to **be attuned to comments from staff nurse about these students.** If these students are not performing their required duties, you will hear about this. As noted in Chapter 3, students and the clinical instructor are guests in the unit. Thus any tasks not completed by the student will be reported by the staff personnel to the nurse manager, who will then immediately notify you. Many instructors are not happy receiving a phone call about a missed task. Therefore communicate clearly and early with your students about their responsibilities.

Another word of caution about the "not-so-high fliers." They may also be those students who are habitually late in leaving the clinical site. That is, at the end of the clinical day, students usually gather at one spot to walk to their conference site for postconference, or they independently meet at a designated time and location for postconference. The at-risk student may lag behind one day and then the next and then the next. When it happens once, try to get the cause for the lateness—maybe a patient had an unexpected test or, for a home visit, maybe the client was unavailable. If it happens repeatedly, it is a cause for concern. A similar finding for this student is that he or she may be the one that other students gathered around. This may just be a casual student gathering, but this can also mean that the "not-so-high flier" has asked for and is receiving assistance from the peers in answering questions.

If you need extra help monitoring some of the students, ask the staff. **Seeking the staff's input is always a wise move,** as it may or may not validate the traits that you see in the student. More frequently though, the staff will come and inform you who they think are your higher level students. Unsolicited feedback about your students is a normal aspect of the clinical teaching arena.

To summarize, if you spot a "not-so-high flier" in your clinical group, just keep an eye on them! No further action is needed on your part. You will be too busy with the normal day's tasks to do anything else with these students, unless of course, a problem occurs. The instructor may continue to observe unsatisfactory behavior. If you are seeing more "red flags" and are unsure about them, review Chapter 10. If more than one "flag" is identified, the instructor is now warned that the student is in jeopardy of clinical course failure. A more elaborate listing of these behaviors are identified in Chapter 10.

Fast facts in a nutshell

- Not-so-high fliers may be difficult to spot.
- High fliers are prepared and assertive.
- Be open to the staff's input regarding certain students.

Part IV

The Performance
Appraisals

Clinical Evaluations

Chapter 8

Making the Most of Student Self-Evaluation

INTRODUCTION

In some programs, students are required to rate their own performance based on the objectives set by the program or the clinical instructor. Students may need assistance in understanding how to effectively complete a self-evaluation. These evaluations are important, as they provide the nursing instructor with a blueprint to use in communicating concepts to students, who in turn will be better prepared to accurately assess their own performance.

In this chapter you will learn:

1. The nature and purpose of student self-evaluations.
2. Suggestions for the instructor to use in guiding students toward a realistic evaluation.

STUDENT PERFORMANCE EVALUATION

One of the most important aspects of clinical care coordination is evaluation (Potter & Perry, 2001). This principle logically extends to evaluation of care rendered by nursing students. Careful explanation of the clinical evaluation tool, including specific examples, should occur at the outset to clearly establish the expectations you will have of your students as they navigate through their clinical experiences. Emphasize to your students that **performance evaluations will be an ongoing process** throughout their nursing careers.

EVALUATION PROCEDURES

Once hired by the nursing program, your initial orientation to the clinical instructor role should include a **detailed explanation of the procedure used to evaluate each student's clinical performance.** This is comparable to the first day in the traditional classroom, when the teacher reviews the course syllabus and details the method by which the course grade will be determined. Various nursing clinical evaluation tools involve "grading." Others are based on "the pass/fail" model. Chapter 11 describes the differences and the challenges of both models, along with examples of each.

STUDENT SELF-EVALUATION

Regardless of what type of evaluation tool is employed, **most nursing programs require students to perform a self-evalu-**

ation. Usually, students submit their self-appraisal a few days before the planned evaluation from the instructor. Senior students with six or more days of clinical instruction, may also be required to submit a self-evaluation for their mid-term. A mid-term evaluation enables the instructor to recognize good performance and facilitate remedial action where needed. Refer to the "Early Warning System" (Chapter 10) for a more detailed explanation of the merits of a mid-term evaluation.

According to Gaberson and Oermann (1999), **development of self-evaluation skills is paramount** for nurses. Because nurses must be competent in a practice that evolves daily management of patient's illnesses and the skillful use of pharmacological therapies and lifesaving equipment, it is essential that nurses continuously self-monitor their performances. Throughout their careers, nurses must determine when they need more education or skill training. It is important, therefore, to foster the development of self-evaluation skill in the student nurse.

SAMPLE GRADING METHODOLOGY

The sample student evaluation grading methodology illustrated in Exhibit 8.1 can be shared with your students on the clinical orientation day. This example is suited for clinical evaluations that are in a graded format.

Many students report that the process of self-evaluation can be anxiety provoking. While this may be true, mild anxiety can promote personal growth. The discussion that ensues once the instructor examines, reviews, and responds to the

EXHIBIT 8.1   Student Self-Evaluation of
Clinical Performance

Grading Methodology

Grading for performance at the clinical site will follow the (*course name or number can appear here*) evaluation tool.

This self-evaluation is your opportunity to comment on your clinical performance. The grade range is a 1 to 5 Likert scale, which is defined as follows:

> 1 – Does not meet clinical criteria
> 2 – Is inconsistent in meeting clinical criteria
> 3 – Meets clinical criteria
> 4 – Exceeds clinical criteria
> 5 – Far exceeds clinical criteria.

Example Objective:
"Attend each clinical session and submit required materials."

If your daily performance and submitted materials meet the expected standard, you may assign yourself a 3. If you exceed these minimum requirements, you may award yourself a 4 or 5, but you must provide *written* evidence for this elevated grade. Keep a log of any instances where you performed above criteria. You cannot rate yourself higher than a 3 if you do not provide the written evidence for that grade. Submit this evidence with your self-evaluation. In the context of this example, here are some ways to exceed clinical criteria and achieve a grade above 3:

• Arrive on the unit early to read your client's chart to ask pertinent questions at the 7 AM preconference.

(continued)

- Submit more than the minimum requirement of one journal per week. Incorporate classroom objectives and knowledge.
- Present a clinically related topic of interest to peers or a client.
- Conduct independent research regarding your client's care.

Please note: Self-evaluation grades higher than 3 that are not supported with written evidence of accomplishment will be reduced to 3.

---

students' self-evaluation can be invaluable. It teaches the student how to accept constructive criticism and provides specific feedback and data on her performance. If a mid-term evaluation is possible, an action plan can be developed for the remainder of the course.

Many **students are seeking feedback and suggestions** in their ongoing pursuit of competency in clinical nursing. This evaluation time can be one of the most important sessions of their entire nursing curriculum. Many of today's experienced nurses can recite an instance where a clinical instructor gave them positive or negative feedback during a clinical evaluation and the impact of that situation on their nursing careers.

Fast facts in a nutshell

- Student self-evaluation is a valuable tool.
- Guidelines are provided to teach students how to document their performances.
- Students self-evaluation, when compared with the instructor's assessment, is an important learning tool.

Chapter 9

The DOs and DON'Ts of
Student Documentation

INTRODUCTION

A common mistake that clinical instructors make in their student clinical evaluations often involves insufficient documentation. "Anecdotal notes" are useful as the traditional format to document clinical performance. However, more official documentation by the clinical instructor becomes imperative when the student's performance leaves her in jeopardy of not passing the course. This chapter illustrates examples of anecdotal notes. It also offers concrete directions on the type of data needed to document the evaluation in a timely way.

In this chapter, you will learn:

1. How to document "anecdotal notes."
2. Key aspects of documentation pertinent to the clinical instructor.

DOCUMENTING STUDENT PERFORMANCE

The clinical instructor's **assessment of student performance is an ongoing process.** The student's evaluation should reflect a compilation of these observations. Ensuring that the student evaluation presents a fair picture of performance requires avoiding common mistakes of judgment.

THE DON'TS

As a new instructor:

- **DO NOT adopt a casual approach to documenting** a students' clinical performance.
- **DO NOT depend on "remembering"** the specifics of each students' experiences when administering medications, assessing OR teaching clients, interacting with staff or peers, or interacting with you.
- DO NOT think that because the student is hanging an intravenous medication or inserting a urinary catheter for their first time, mistakes should be disregarded because of a lack of preparation.
- DO NOT conclude that little harm or injury will ensue after a student encounter, such as patient assessment with a client, even though the nurse stated that the client was "upset" that day.
- **DO NOT assume that the instructor has no financial or legal risk** associated with student errors because students carry their own liability insurance.

THE DOS

A casual approach to documenting student clinical performance can lead to a final student evaluation that cannot be supported. The instructor may "feel" that a student adequately performed during a specific rotation, but did not exceed the minimum expectation of the clinical program. That student may, quite possibly, have an entirely different perspective. The student may believe that she performed in an exemplary manner and can cite specific examples in her self-evaluation. Unless the instructor has maintained an organized file of "anecdotal notes" to refute this perception, the instructor's assessment may face a student challenge that can often involve extensive follow-up and work by the instructor. This may include discussions between the instructor and the level coordinator or school chairperson, as well as other assigned faculty members. There are usually procedures in place regarding these types of student issues. Each nursing program has a different procedure for handling student clinical course issues.

If an instructor depends on "remembering" the specifics of each student's experience, the student evaluation can be murky and irrelevant. With as many as ten students to evaluate, even a person with a sharp memory may have difficulty recalling the specifics of each student's performance and implementation of various nursing skills in ten different areas of the unit.

In evaluating students, **never disregard "lack of preparation."** If students have been notified that they will be administering medications and performing certain procedures, it is incumbent on the students to prepare by practicing in the nursing lab. Clinical instructors often have minimal time to teach and review an entire procedure for a student, particularly if the client is to receive treatment in a timely manner. Nursing labs are available in all nursing programs today. It is the students' responsibility to make arrangements to visit the lab to review necessary skills before their clinical experiences.

Make the nursing staff your ally. They have eyes and ears that can interpret and gather more information about your students' performance than you can obtain alone. If a nurse or nursing assistant mentions to you that a patient or his family seemed upset after the student performed a skill or entered a client room, INVESTIGATE. This revelation often is a "red flag" that indicates a possible problem for the student, the school of nursing, and YOU. Go into the patient's room, introduce yourself to the patient and family, and ask how the student interaction was received by the client. It is better to take care of any potential problem immediately rather than let it fester. Addressing it a week or two later may mean the difference between a prompt resolution and a legal situation.

FINANCIAL LIABILITY

Understand your financial liability at the clinical site. Teachers and students are held to the same standards of care that a reasonably prudent person with the same level of education and experience would use in the same or similar circumstances (Gaberson & Oermann, 1999). According to Gaberson and Oermann, a specific criterion is used to determine a teacher's liability for an act deemed negligent by a student.

Teachers are not liable for negligent acts performed by their students if they have done the following:

1. **Selected appropriate learning activities** based on skills necessary to complete their assignment.
2. **Determined that the students have the necessary knowledge and skills** to complete the assignment.
3. **Provided necessary guidance.**

Yes, your students do have liability insurance, but you too are liable if the aforementioned standards are not in place when your student performs an unsafe act. As an instructor, it is prudent to carry liability insurance. Check with national nursing organizations, which can provide further information about liability insurance for educators. You can also check with the chairperson or head of your nursing program for this information.

ANECDOTAL NOTES

Each day, the instructor will have students assume an assignment (as detailed in Part VI). **Devise a system for maintaining "anecdotal notes"** relating to each student's performance, perhaps by simply filing them with each day's assignment paper in a binder for the entire rotation. Your own notes during the day will help jog your memory when it is time to conduct the clinical evaluation. You may also want to maintain a book with a separate pages for each student—a copybook of sorts. After each clinical day, jot down a few notes about each student. An example of such a note might be:

Mary administered Ancef I.V. and gave three oral medications to her patient. Her knowledge base of the oral medications was weak. I recommended to her that she write down pertinent facts about the meds before she contacts me saying she is prepared to give meds.

Writing such brief notes will help you identify whether a specific student followed your suggestion or repeated the same weak performance the next time that she administered meds. If a particular student repeated the same substandard performance, it could be a "warning" sign. Discussion of warning signs for clinical instructors can be found in Chapter 10.

Any system that you are comfortable with will do. Even an electronic record of this information is effective. The bottom line is that **you need to write a note or two on each student each day of the clinical rotation,** so take the time to document. The nursing profession teaches new students that if it is not documented, it did not happen. For a successful student evaluation, make sure that your anecdotal notes reveal what did happen.

Fast facts in a nutshell

- Avoid the "mistakes" of a new clinical instructor by documenting student performance.
- Anecdotal notes are paramount to all instructors.
- Written recordings of clinical performance are needed to support documenting a student's weakness or failure.

Chapter 10

Early Warning System

INTRODUCTION

Many experienced clinical nursing instructors use a large amount of intuition when observing students. There are usually warning signs if a student is in jeopardy of not meeting the clinical objectives of the course. For example, a student may perform a nursing skill in a certain manner or communicate an aspect of the nursing process in such a way that the experienced instructor is alerted to a potential problem. Because nurses are charged with serious and potentially life-sustaining responsibilities, these sometimes subtle "warning signs" are important to heed and address.

In this chapter, you will learn:

1. How to identify the warning signs that a student may be in jeopardy of not passing or safely performing in the clinical setting.
2. Important tips to develop a "sixth sense," or intuition, to help determine which students are at risk for performing unsafe practices on patients.

EARLY WARNING SIGNS

As stated in Chapter 8, a **mid-term evaluation is recommended** for any clinical rotation that extends for at least six days. If the rotation is fewer than six days, a mid-term evaluation is difficult to adequately complete. However, an informal meeting between you and the student may be prudent. The informal meeting might be as simple as a quick review of the evaluation form and your observations of the student to date. The meeting also may offer you the opportunity to discuss any early warning signs that you have observed in the student's performance.

CLINICAL OBJECTIVES

Assessing student performance at the clinical site can be a formidable task. The nursing instructor is not afforded the luxury of objective testing to measure student success. There is no fill-in-the-blank means of gauging the student's knowledge and safety on the floor, nor is there a multiple choice test that can measure clinical effectiveness. Rather, the clinical teacher must base his or her judgment on direct observation within the context of written clinical objectives whose lack of precision can make them challenging to interpret. Examples of clinical objectives include the following:

- Demonstrates **ability to meet the psychological needs** of the critically ill client.
- Interprets own **verbal and nonverbal communications** accurately.
- Demonstrates **appropriate interactions** with all patients.

Different nursing instructors can interpret these objectives in various ways. How does a novice clinical instructor decide what information to note for later use in evaluating student performance in terms of the program's objectives?

"RED FLAG" WARNINGS

There is another aspect to becoming an astute clinical instructor. This involves **awareness of the more common "red flags"** that students may wave during their clinical rotation – signals that warrant an instructor's observation, concern, consultation, and action plan.

Here are some examples of "warning signs":

- **Hedging:** Students who arrive unprepared sometimes will try to answer your questions by hesitantly bringing up many unrelated facts. An example of "hedging" is when the instructor asks the student to explain why the client has intermittent compression devices on his legs after surgery. The student replies that it is for post-op prevention of complications, but cannot specifically describe what complication and how these devices actually prevent complication. If the students do not know the specifics of why a nursing measure is taken, they cannot evaluate the effectiveness of the measure.
- **Late submission of assignments:** Students are given a timetable for completing their journals and other assigned paperwork. Students who submit this paperwork late (more than one time) may be having difficulty. They may be working too many hours at a job to complete their work in a timely manner. They may not be conscious of the need for timeliness

in a field where it is necessary to be on time with nursing care. Late assignment submissions often have a cause that you as the instructor should investigate. Do not just think that you are helping the student by "letting it go." The vital importance that the timely completion of tasks plays in the care of the patient must be instilled at the outset.

• **Late arrival at the clinical site:** Nursing is an ongoing process in which the arriving nurse continues the flow of care rendered by her predecessor from the preceding shift. Lateness can greatly compromise this continuity. Students must clearly understand that being late for the clinical is much more serious than being late for class. Unless the lateness is an unavoidable and isolated instance, such as a car accident, failure to appear at the designated hour is a very disconcerting sign. Do they really appreciate the tremendous responsibilities that accompany this field? Are other parts of their lives interfering with their education? Whatever the cause, it is the instructor's job to address the situation with the student, develop consequences for any continued lateness, and evaluate the student's ability to continue in nursing.

• **Performing skills without supervision:** Chapter 4 provided information about orientation day for an instructor and new students. It was stated that the rules and requirements of the host facility, school, and instructor should be provided in writing and reviewed. Noted in this review would be the instruction that "no nursing skill should be performed or medication given by the student without supervision. " The instructor should clearly state who can provide such supervision. Will it always be you, or are there circumstances when the professional nurse in your organization may supervise the student? Some instructors require that the students sign a statement at orientation day that they understand these requirements. Incorporate this prudent practice in your own clinical oversight, because a student who performs a task or skill without the appropriate supervision can cause a serious and potentially deadly error. Should a breach of the supervision rule occur, it is paramount that you act immediately! Have a conference with the student that day, if possible right after the incident. You usually need to report this error to the unit floor manager and your supervisor at the school of nursing (clinical level coordinator). Follow the school's policies in this regard (see Chapter 2) and also be aware of its "Safe Practice" criteria (see Chapter 17).

• **Chronic personal crises:** Every instructor knows that "life happens." Anyone can have a bad day or perform in a manner that is not optimal. At the same time, be aware of the student who continually offers excuses for less than stellar clinical performance. For example, all students may be advised by the instructor to visit their nursing lab before clinical to review certain procedures, such as insulin injections or administering medications through a feeding tube. If you notice that a particular student clearly does not know which step to take first to perform this required skill, clearly the student's preparation was not adequate. The student may offer reasons for poor performance, ranging from physical illness to emotional heartbreak. At first, many instructors will extend the benefit of the doubt and walk the student through the procedure. This forgiving approach, however, should include advising the student that the lack of preparation indicates that more review time is warranted with the lab coordinator and should be accompanied by appropriate documentation in the anecdotal notes. However, if you observe the same lack of preparation in the same student a second time, you have received a "warning sign."

TAKING ACTION ON WARNING SIGNS

What should the clinical instructor do about these "warning signs"? If you are relatively new to the field of clinical instruction, **discuss these observations with a more experienced colleague.** Instructors develop their own methodologies for working with students. Courtesy would indicate that you notify the lab instructor in advance as to what you expect from the lab time. You may then send the student to the nursing lab with a written instruction of what happened in clinical. You may request a written note or e-mail notification from the lab instructor confirming that the student did indeed complete the requested lab time. If enough "warning signs" accrue, the student may be in jeopardy of failing the clinical course. Familiarize yourself with the performance evaluation form and follow some of the suggestions in documenting unsafe practice in Chapters 9 and 17.

IMPORTANCE OF INTUITION

As you become a more experienced clinical instructor, you will rely more on your intuition. A student will impress you with some of her interactions with patients, and you will realize that you need not observe that student as keenly as others. With as many as ten students, you need to develop a sense

for determining which students need close scrutiny for patient safety and which are more competent in their skills.

Trust your instincts. You developed these similar instincts as a staff or primary nurse when you "just had a feeling" that the client was not doing well, and you spent additional time with that patient. It will be the same with student
nurses. In time, your own instincts will alert you to the students who have a greater potential of possibly causing injury
to the clients in their care.

Fast facts in a nutshell

- Be alert for "warning signs" in students' performance.
- If you observe a "warning sign," document it, and
  seek advice when needed.
- Trust your instincts concerning "problem students."

Chapter 11

Graded Clinical vs. Pass/Fail Evaluations

INTRODUCTION

The time constraint inherent in clinical teaching has been acknowledged in this book. This is what makes the job of clinical instructors a bit more challenging then other faculty in academia. However, because the profession of nursing is seen as a practice discipline at its core, students must be evaluated according to how they practice and, therefore, "perform." Clinical students can be graded with a pass/fail, a satisfactory/unsatisfactory, a letter/number grade, or a combination of these systems.

In this chapter, you will learn:

1. How each grading system works.
2. The advantages and disadvantages of each system.

GRADING STUDENTS

In clinical teaching, the **evaluation is the most difficult and emotionally charged responsibility** (Scanlan, Care, & Gressler, 2001). Clinical instructors must deal with degrees of subjectivity in evaluating another person's performance, as well as with the fact that they do not have much time to spend with, let alone evaluate, students!

Challenges in Evaluating Students

Clinical instructors are consistently faced with several challenges in evaluating student performance. In some programs, an entire clinical rotation may last only two weeks. Moreover, the instructor is responsible for not just one student, but a group of students! For example, in a generic nursing program, the clinical instructor may be responsible for written evaluations and grades for as many as ten students after a seven week medical surgical rotation.

Knowledge of Course Objectives

Instructors **observe and score a student's performance based on a set of critical criteria linked to the course objectives.** Therefore, it is imperative that clinical instructors familiarize themselves with the clinical course objectives, set clinical evaluation periods and, most importantly, the grading system.

Unanticipated Events

In addition, anticipated and unanticipated events can affect the valuable time instructors have with students. For most clinical rotations, the first day is usually the assigned hospital orientation day. Other days may be lost to university or nursing program events that students are required to attend or legal holidays on which classes are canceled. Unanticipated events, such as extreme weather conditions or school disasters, may result in school closure. All of these events affect the number of days instructors have for observing and evaluating student performance.

TYPES OF GRADING SYSTEMS

The grading system for clinical courses is primarily based on the student's achievement of certain course objectives. Clinical courses are usually offered on a pass/fail grading system or letter/number grading system. See Exhibit 11.1 for a commonly used grading system that could be found in any student handbook.

Pass/fail grades and satisfactory/unsatisfactory grades are similar and do not provide comparative gradations among passing students. **A letter grade offers a finer evaluation** of a student's performance. Grading is usually specific to the nursing program. Exhibit 11.2 is another example of a grading system that would be found in a clinical course.

EXHIBIT 11.1   Grading System

The grading system used for nursing courses is based on the student's achievement of the course objectives. The grading scale is as follows:

Theory course

Letter Grade	Percentage Grade	*Quality Points
A	93–100	4.0
B	84–92	3.0
C	75–83	2.0
F	Below 75	0.0

Clinical Laboratory:

S = Satisfactory
U = Unsatisfactory

Satisfactory or Unsatisfactory

Clinical laboratory is graded as satisfactory or unsatisfactory. A final grade of satisfactory is required in the clinical component of a nursing course. If the student is not demonstrating a pattern of satisfactory clinical performance, the clinical instructor will meet with the student to formulate a plan for improvement. Students must achieve all clinical course objectives/competencies by the end of the course to receive a satisfactory grade. An unsatisfactory clinical grade at the end of the course results in course failure regardless of grades received on classroom assignments, tests, and examinations. The final course grade will be recorded as an F.

EXHIBIT 11.2   NSG 411 Advanced Adaptation Course

NSL 411 Clinical Course

Laboratory component Grading System

The grading system used for nursing clinical courses is based on the student's achievement of the course objectives. The grading scale is as follows:

Pass or Fail

Clinical laboratory is graded as pass or fail. This means that you will not receive a letter grade for the course; rather you will receive a grade of "P" for satisfactory work and "F" for unsatisfactory work. Pass grades are included in total credits earned but pass/fail grades are not included in the grade point average.

CLINICAL EVALUATION FORMS

Clinical evaluation forms reflect the specific behavioral objectives of that course. To assist students in meeting these objectives, specific clinical criteria are established and written out clearly on the evaluation form. These clinical criteria are presented to the students and discussed with them at the first clinical day. The student's performance and the instructor's observations are the key elements in the evaluation process.

Evaluations of clinical criteria are clearly highlighted in the clinical evaluation tool and may be given orally to the student by the instructor during the evaluation time.

An example of a clinical objective is:

The student applies knowledge of medical surgical nursing when providing patient care.

For this objective, an instructor using the pass/fail grading system would report a P (Pass) or an F (Fail) for this objective based on that student's performance in the setting. In a program using the letter/number grading system, the clinical evaluation tool would include a rating scale. Thus, for this objective, the instructor would score the student based on the rating scale. The scale is usually a Likert-type scale ranging from 1 to 5. It is to that highlighted in Chapter 8. The scale scores for each objective would then be tallied to give a final clinical score.

Fast facts in a nutshell

- Each program defines its own clinical evaluation system.
- Clinical objectives are highlighted in the clinical evaluation tool.
- A 1 to 5 rating scale is found in a letter/number grading system.

Part V

Communication at
Clinical Conferences

Chapter 12

Preconferences

INTRODUCTION

Preconferences are preclinical meetings held at the start of the clinical day. The conference is led by the instructor and can provide teaching and learning opportunities. These occur because the clinical instructor has the opportunity to assess the student's preparation and assignment for the clinical day and to observe key aspects of the student's communication skills that are necessary to nursing practice. Communication competence is an essential nursing skill because of the daily interactions nurses have with patients and other healthcare providers. Proper preparation for the clinical day is also essential and is an evaluation objective for all levels of nursing students.

In this chapter you will learn:

1. The value and proper use of preconference time.
2. The role of the preconference in relation to the objectives of the nursing process. One scenario of a type of preconference will be highlighted.

WHAT IS A PRECONFERENCE?

During the clinical rotations, the instructor will schedule conferences. These conferences are usually held before the start of a clinical day and are called a preconference. If scheduled at the end of the day, they are called postconferences. For the clinical faculty, **these conferences are a teaching learning strategy** because they are expected to follow-up on elements from the classroom lectures. They also **use these conferences to plan learning opportunities for their students.** Among nurse educators, this is referred to as "the application of theory into practice."

STUDENT GUIDANCE

Each clinical instructor should remember that no one else is giving these students direction about the specific clinical rotation. Instructors are responsible for providing all guidance and addressing all questions regarding all aspects of the clinical experience. Their job responsibilities include setting the rules and structuring the clinical day according to the objectives of the program. Although students should learn the majority of the rules and instructor expectations at the orientation day, conferences with students during the rotation also provide opportunities to share expectations and reinforce clinical guidelines.

Daily Expectations

Students will become frustrated if they do not know what is expected of them each clinical day. Students should not be surprised about the rules and guidelines nor should they arrive at a clinical unit without adequate preparation from the instructor. What kind of "preparation" is the clinical instructor responsible for? The instructor must "prepare" the students for his or her expectations and what is expected of their performance. This requires clarifying the clinical objectives set forth by the nursing program, which are usually broad and unspecific in relation to the actual elements of patient care. **Each student needs to know the specific elements of patient care for which he or she will be responsible** and the general timeline of each clinical day. This can best be done during a preconference.

Patient Care Assignments

The students usually receive their patient care assignments at this time. If they received their patient assignment before the preconference, the clinical instructor can review each student's plan of care during the preconference. In essence, the **purposes** of a preconference are to give faculty an opportunity to **prepare the students** for the clinical day, to **review any work** from the students, and to **set the structure of the clinical day** to avoid frustration for all parties. An example of a preconference scenario is provided in Exhibit 12.1.

EXHIBIT 12.1   Preconference Scenario

At the orientation day, Jason, the clinical instructor, informed students that at the beginning of each clinical day, at 6:30 AM sharp, he will hold a preconference with the group in the cafeteria meeting room. The purpose was to give them the three learning goals for the clinical day, as well as to give each of them their patient care assignment. At one particular preconference, Jason shared the following goals for students to fulfill on that clinical day: (1) to complete an assessment on their patient; (2) to document that assessment and (3) to understand the medication list for each patient. Students were given these goals orally and on a written handout from the instructor. In addition, one student, Nancy, received a client in room 550, a 10-year-old patient with cystic fibrosis. The clinical instructor then directed Nancy and all the students to review the disease and its medical and nursing management during the rest of the preconference time.

In some programs, clinical instructors are expected to visit the agency in advance of the clinical day to review and select patients for students, so that students can receive patient care assignments before the clinical day. If this is the expectation of your nursing program, then the preconference format may be structured differently than the scenario above. The preconference time can then be used to evaluate the student's understanding of a patient's disease and medical management and to assess adequate student preparation for the clinical day. **The preconference time can also be used as a teaching opportunity.** The nursing instructor may highlight a certain class of medications, such as salicylates, and have the students discuss its interactions and side effects. In addition, student communication skills may also be observed and evaluated. The instructor can inform students that preconference time will begin with each student verbalizing their patient's initials, the diagnosis, medical and nursing management, and nursing goals.

When students receive patient care assignments in advance of the clinical day, the expectations are a bit different. There are higher expectations at the preconference and postconference because the students have more resources and time to prepare for the clinical day. Thus, the **manner in which patient care assignments are distributed plays a role in the structure of the preconference session.** However, throughout the clinical rotation, clinical faculty use these preconference sessions as evaluation opportunities to assess the student's clinical day preparation and review their knowledge of the nursing process.

Fast facts in a nutshell

- The clinical nursing preconference is simply a "preclinical" conference.
- For the clinical instructor, the preconference is a time for teaching and learning opportunities.
- The preconference can also be used to evaluate each student's preparation and assessment of his or her patient assignment.

Chapter 13

Postconferences

INTRODUCTION

Postconferences are held at the conclusion of a clinical day. Students are usually expected to present their patients at the postconference. This time allows the instructor to address any events that may have occurred during the clinical day.

In this chapter you will learn:

1. The purpose of postconferences.
2. An explanation of their importance to the overall learning objectives of the clinical course and the analysis of patient care.

WHAT IS A POSTCONFERENCE?

Preconferences and postconferences are similar. They are both meeting times at which clinical issues are discussed and questions about clinical objectives are answered by the instructor.

However most clinical faculty will lead the preconference, but **follow the students' lead at the postconference.** The reason is primarily associated with the timing of the conference. The conclusion of a long clinical day provides a better opportunity for the instructor to ascertain students' understanding of their patient's care and to question students about their findings from the chart and their own patient assessment.

TEACHING OPPORTUNITIES

Clinical faculty can also **use postconferences as teaching learning opportunities.** As such, the clinical instructor can, for example, review lab values with the clinical group at one postconference session. Or, the postconference can be used to link class theory with actual practice elements. For example, if the class topic is respiratory obstructive disorders, during postconference, the instructor can elaborate on the lab values associated with this class of disorders. Or, the postconference may focus on respiratory acidosis and the role played by arterial blood gases. A postconference can also be a learning opportunity, which can be self-directed learning. For example, the instructor may have students review Internet resources available for teaching about their assigned patient. Most clinical faculty will plan many learning activities for their students. Another such activity is student presentations.

Student Presentations

Students can be assigned a **10-minute presentation on a nursing topic** appropriate to the objectives of the clinical rotation.

These student presentations also can also be viewed as a communication assignment. Another assigned learning activity can relate to research articles. Depending on the level of the undergraduate student, the clinical instructor can collect literature reviews or have students **verbalize some aspects of a research article** during a postconference. Like a preconference, postconferences can take up to one hour. Because of time limitations, however, students should receive an assigned due date for each learning assignment. Wink (1995) presents many alternative strategies for instructors to try during conferences. Read her article for more ideas.

Understand Conference Limitations

Do not overwhelm the conference time by including too many teaching learning opportunities. Always be true to your students and be in touch with their psychosocial well-being. At the end of a clinical day during which they have been continuously evaluated, they are mentally and physically exhausted. **Know their limits.** This important tip will keep you from being frustrated as you set your own expectations for the postconference.

SHARING STUDENT EXPERIENCES

One word of caution about these conferences. Although clinical faculty can and often do use preconferences and postconferences as an evaluation opportunity, not all conferences should be seen as evaluation time. The effective clinical instructor will also hold conferences that are devoid of the evaluation "hat." These conferences allow students to share experiences and interact with the group without the stress of performance evaluation. Inform your students when they will be specifically evaluated. **Allow for free sharing of experiences.** Once you do that, your conferences will run smoothly and will meet your instructor expectations. If you choose, you can use the first 10 minutes of postconference to ask and discuss an open-ended question, such as "For those who gave medications today, how did you like the experience?

As many teaching and learning opportunities exist, the clinical instructor should be cautioned not to try too many at once. Remember that postconferences can be a productive time for teaching and learning, a time when students have an opportunity to address concerns regarding their patient care or their performance. Students may also question something that happened during the course of a day.

Sample Scenario

Exhibit 13.1 provides an example of an appropriate event to discuss at a postconference. As this exhibit illustrates, the student's assessment findings and the actions by the primary nurse can be a key discussion point for the postconference. In this scenario, the student verbalized key aspects of her patient's condition with the clinical group and shared the events that unfolded during her care of the patient. Students in this clinical group had many questions regarding the patient's diet and whether this could have been a factor related to the hypoglycemia.

EXHIBIT 13.1   Postconference Discussion Point

An undergraduate student in a progressive care unit was caring for a female patient recovering from open heart surgery and the complications of pneumonia. The patient could not speak because of a tracheostomy tube and was breathing on room air. This was the second day the student was assigned to this patient. Knowing the patient from the previous day, the student noticed that the patient seemed more lethargic and became diaphoretic as she was completing the noon vital signs. The clinical instructor observed the student as she reported her findings to the assigned primary nurse. The blood glucose was quickly checked and revealed that the patient was acutely hypoglycemic. The primary nurse then alerted the physician.

Lessons Learned from the Scenario

This example provides many good observation points about this particular student. The student was able to effectively verbalize the event and share her experience with the group. More importantly, the clinical instructor observed her keen assessment of the patient as well as her actions of critical thinking (rechecking vital signs) and then her appropriate reaction (verbalizing her assessment concerns to the primary nurse).

Clinical instructors will find that time is limited during the course of a clinical day to actually stop and teach. The day progresses so quickly that many key events come and go without time to "pause" to share a key aspect of care or highlight a particular intervention. The time to do this is at postconference. When there is something to be emphasized, an item to be taught, or an event to debrief, **postconferences provide the time to share and discuss experiences.**

Fast facts in a nutshell

- Postconference time should not be directed by the instructor. Rather, they are a time to debrief about the aspects of the day.
- Have postconferences without the evaluation hat.
- Postconferences can be used as teaching and learning opportunities.

Part VI

The Art of Making A
Clinical Assignment

Chapter 14

Unplanned Events

INTRODUCTION

As any nurse or professional will tell you, the world of healthcare is filled with unexpected or unanticipated moments. In fact, aside from the nursing process itself, there is nothing "routine" in health and illness. Relay this fact to your students who are expecting to find their same patient in the same condition every day.

Anticipating unplanned events, such as low census, acute changes in a patient condition, resident outings, or client discharges, is key when developing an assignment that will provide the best learning experience for the student.

In this chapter, you will learn:

1. How to anticipate or plan in advance for changes in a student's clinical assignment.
2. How to develop a "toolbox" of potential alternate assignments that will save time when unplanned events occur.

PLANNING ASSIGNMENTS

It is sometimes impossible to predict the census or patient composition of the clinical unit to which your students have been assigned during their rotation. It may also be difficult to predict which clients will be available for your students to interact with at a retirement facility, daycare setting, or school. How can you, as the clinical instructor, plan an assignment for your charges and also ensure that your students are meeting their learning objectives for the clinical course?

First, one has to **create a student nurse clinical assignment.** Think of all of the potential clinical placements in which today's student nurses may find themselves. Students are at nursery schools, senior centers, maternity units, and community settings, just to name a few. Listed below are some standard guidelines that instructor's can use in all settings.

GUIDELINES FOR CLINICAL ASSIGNMENTS

- **Be familiar with the student evaluation tool,** which will list the clinical objectives.
- **Use this tool as your "roadmap"** for developing assignments.
- **Develop a relationship with the nursing staff** at your facility so its members can assist you.
- **Accept the nursing staff's hints and suggestions.** Their input is invaluable. For example, a staff nurse may tell you, "that patient is not good for a student." HEED THEIR ADVICE. They know. They will know what client has an anxious family that would be hesitant to allow a student

nurse to care for its relative. They will also know the patient who is be too threatening for a novice student.

- **Arrive the day or evening before,** if the unit allows. If not, at least arrive earlier than your nursing students.
- **Inquire at the nursing report** (transfer of information about residents/clients from one shift to the on-coming shift) about clients who would appreciate a student and learn the client's schedule for that day. Will the client be off of the unit most of the day for tests? Are they in too much pain to talk with the student on a day when a primary objective is oral communication?
- **Avoid writing down all of the patient data.** It is not your role to communicate this detailed level of information to the student. Part of the learning experience—and an essential component of your evaluation of each student—will be the student's understanding of what information is essential and where to locate that information. See Appendix C for a sample tool that can be used to e-mail brief data to students the day before the clinical. Ensure that patient confidentiality is maintained when communicating via e-mail. This means that no patient name is allowed. Room numbers or just initials may be used.
- **Be cognizant of each student's strengths and weaknesses.** For example, a student who has some initial self-confidence issues may not be the one to take on the cantankerous senior who will "order" her around all day. The older student with a greater sense of herself would be the appropriate student for this challenging client. Students who are able to handle more difficult clients may appropriately receive a higher grade than others.

- **Be flexible.** The most detailed and well-prepared assignment may fall apart when clients are not available on the scheduled day or are unable to accept a student for some reason. A sense of humor will serve you well on these days.

UNPLANNED EVENTS

Here is the irony. Although events are unplanned, you can be sure they will occur. **Try to have a "back-up" plan** when creating a student assignment. This can be accomplished by carrying with you relevant clinical case studies to use if circumstances result in a student's inability to complete objectives on a given day. For example, the student may have planned to perform her psychosocial assessment on her assigned resident, but that resident has unexpectedly left for the day. The staff states that no other resident is available, so the student and resident have agreed to complete the assessment on the following day. This is an opportune time to give the student the case studies you are carrying, with the objective of reviewing and then presenting them to her peers at a postconference.

Another example of an unplanned event could be the student who is overwhelmed halfway into the shift. She shares her fear that the client's needs will not be met that day during her scheduled time with the client. You can always assign a second student to provide assistance. Often, that student will be the one who is able to complete most of her responsibilities more quickly than the others. Working together teaches students that helping one another is essential to the practice of nursing. **Often, students learn best from a**

peer. The peer can teach the slower student some "tricks of the trade" in a nonthreatening manner that is beneficial to all. As you detect differences in the students' abilities, capture your observations in the anecdotal notes, as mentioned in Chapter 9.

ALTERNATIVE ASSIGNMENTS

Lastly, develop a list of "alternative assignments" that can be employed with your students when needed. Chapter 15 will describe in detail what is meant by "alternative assignments."

Fast facts in a nutshell

- Preparation for student assignments often will prove beneficial.
- Unplanned events will occur despite your best plans.
- Flexibility and a positive relationship with the staff at your facility will assist you in adapting a student assignment.

Chapter 15

Alternative Assignments

INTRODUCTION

All levels of students (from first to final year) will benefit from assignments "outside" of the specified clinical rotation. Supplemental experience in a department other than their assigned one enhances the educational value of the clinical site. This alternative assignment can occur in the community, pediatric, maternity, psychiatric, or medical-surgical rotations of a student's clinical experience.

As noted in Chapter 14, it is helpful to have a plan for the "unplanned events" that inevitably will occur on many clinical days. This chapter presents samples of alternative assignments based on the particular clinical rotations. They are accompanied by tips on methods for coordinating and cultivating these alternative assignments to be benefit all parties, but especially the students.

In this chapter, you will learn:

1. The value of providing alternative assignments for your students

2. Sample alternative assignments for many different clinical rotations that instructors can select for immediate use in their current work.

MEETING PROGRAM OBJECTIVES

In all types of nursing programs—associate, diploma, or baccalaureate—the "guiding light" of your clinical rotations are the clinical objectives specified on the evaluation tool. Some schools use generic objectives that can be applied to multiple locations, such as maternity, pediatric, or psychiatric nursing settings. Other schools may have different objectives for each specific rotation. No matter what the evaluation tool, the instructor's must follow these objectives and **plan opportunities for all of students to meet each program objective.** This is often challenging. Remember that you may have up to ten students in your rotation, and each must be given an equal opportunity to meet the required objectives.

ALTERNATIVE ASSIGNMENTS

For this reason, it is prudent to **develop "alternative assignments" for each clinical rotation.** These alternative assignments serve many purposes. They offer a chance to carry the stated purpose and knowledge of this rotation to a different location, where the student can often interact with different staff personnel. Another purpose of these alternative assignments is to **create a more manageable number of students** for you to evaluate and supervise on any given day. For example, an instructor has ten students on an acute pediatric hospital unit to supervise. Several of these students need to administer medications, and all need to complete comprehensive patient care. This is a formidable task for any instructor. If two or three alternative assignments were created that met some of the clinical objective of this pediatric rotation, then the instructor would have only seven nursing students on the acute care floor instead of ten.

Appropriate Assignments

An important caveat to these alternative assignments is that they need to facilitate the students' attempts to meet their clinical objectives and that the level coordinator needs to agree with your assessment of this alternative as safe and beneficial. An example of how these assignments can be abused or deemed inappropriate is shown in Exhibit 15.1.

EXHIBIT 15.1   Inappropriate Alternative Assignment

Megan, a new nursing clinical instructor supervised nine students for a four-day rotation through an acute psychiatric unit. At an orientation session, the level coordinator communicated the clinical objectives to this instructor. The school has used this site for many years, and the school and unit nurses had a good working relationship.

(continued)

Megan decided unilaterally that nine students were too many to supervise at one site. Without asking the level coordinator, she asked the facility's emergency room (ER) if she could send two students to the ER each of the three clinical days and three students on a fourth day. All would therefore have the same opportunity.

The students reported this practice to the level coordinator. They were concerned about missing the needed opportunity to observe patients and meet their assigned objectives with them on an acute psychiatric unit. Because this was only a four-day rotation, their concern was well founded. They all enjoyed the ER experience but knew that they were not meeting their primary objectives.

The level coordinator called the new instructor, reprimanded her, and instructed her to keep all students on the acute psychiatric unit as prescribed by the nursing curriculum. Megan was asked why she had assigned these students to an alternative placement like the ER during their brief psychiatric rotation. She responded that she thought students would have an opportunity to observe clients who came to the ER when in acute psychiatric crisis. While there was a possibility that this could occur, it was unlikely. Moreover, Megan needed to check with her level coordinator before any alternative assignment was created.

With the above example in mind, remember that while alternative assignments can and often are beneficial, they must adhere to the clinical objectives of the rotation and must receive the the level coordinator's approval. Table 15.1 illustrates some possible alternative assignments for students in different rotations. Each instructor needs to modify these suggestions to his or her own school's specifications and requirements.

Clinical Rotation Assignments

TABLE 15.1	Samples of possible alternative assignments
Clinical rotation	Alternative assignment
Acute hospital pediatric floor	Day with a pediatric nurse practitioner
Maternity rotation in hospital	Visit to a free-standing birth center
Acute psychiatric rotation	Visit to an outpatient community mental health center
Medical–surgical floor	Day in the critical care unit
Community health	Day at a migrant farm location

These are only a few of the creative and valuable alternative assignments that you can have in your repertoire. You must also give students clear instructions with each alternative assignment. For example, the student who spends the day with the pediatric nurse practitioner during his pediatric rotation must have a written format with objectives and requirements for that day.

Importance of Feedback

A written assignment describing how each of the above objectives were or were not fulfilled during that student's day may be required. It is also advisable to **get feedback from the nurse practitioner about the student's performance.** Exhibit 15.2 provides an example of instructions for an alternative assignment.

EXHIBIT 15.2   Assignments for Clinical Rotations

During your experience with the pediatric nurse practitioner, you will be concentrating on objectives 1, 2, and 3 of your evaluation tool, which read:

1. Observe the role of each nurse in his or her relationship to ill children and in performing nursing responsibilities.

2. Familiarize yourself with the Nurse Practice Act and observe the nurse's extended role as a practitioner.

3. Assess the nursing process used with each pediatric client during your experience.

Some examples of negative feedback would be:

"The student just sat in the corner of the office and read through journals."

"I attempted to engage the student and often pointed out different assessment findings, but she just looked, said little, and returned to her corner seat."

This feedback is invaluable. This data could alert you to one of the "early warning signals" mentioned in Chapter 10. What is interfering with a student's ability to learn? Is it lack of motivation? Lack of sleep? Something is amiss, and it is now your opportunity to address the problem and try to correct it.

It is important that students do not view an alternative assignment as a "day off." Convey this information by carefully orienting students as to the goals and written assignment for the day. Let the student know that you will talk to the nurses at the alternative assignment and receive feedback.

Prepare the Clinical Setting

As the clinical instructor, it is important to "scope" out the alternative assignment site and experience it for yourself before assigning a student. Verify that the nursing staff is willing to teach and have a student "shadow" them for the day. Be clear with the staff and management about the specifics of the student's assignment. For example, if the student is spending the day with the pediatric nurse practitioner, make sure that the student does not assess or document or perform any procedure while at the site. The student would probably not be covered for any liability if in a different locale or part of the clinical rotation. Stress that this is an observation experience only and be very clear with your students about the parameters of their responsibilities on that day.

Individualizing Student Assignments

While there are general rules or guidelines for each chapter of this book as they pertain to student education, **each student's**

clinical experience needs to be individualized. For example, perhaps a student is struggling on the assigned unit. He may have made a medication error or missed an important client assessment. Under these circumstances, carefully consider the appropriateness of giving the student an alternative assignment. You may not be able to observe this student at that assignment, and he may need more time to meet the objectives on your specific unit. If this is true, do not send this student to the alternative assignment. Inform the student why this is occurring. Explain that you need more intensive time to observe his performance and that he needs more opportunity to master the objectives of this specific clinical site. Informing your level coordinator is again a wise step in case the student complains to the level head about this change.

It is also imperative that instructors document the "Why" and "How" of this decision. Refer to Chapter 9 on how to document the performance of a student who is at risk of failing.

Fast facts in a nutshell

- Alternative assignments serve many practical purposes.
- These assignments must be meaningful and approved.
- Specific clinical objectives must be established for each alternative assignment, with written and oral feedback from the student.

Part VII

Competencies Not Met

Chapter 16

Punctuality and Absences

INTRODUCTION

Each clinical course runs for a specific number of clinical hours and days, so that competencies are maintained. Students are required to arrive on time and be present each and every clinical day. Absences and tardiness affect the performance of students and must be monitored closely by the clinical instructor.

In this chapter, you will learn:

1. The impact of absences and lateness on meeting clinical objectives.
2. A summary of the set policies written concerning clinical absences and tardiness.

BASIC COMPETENCIES IN THE
CLINICAL SETTING

The student is assigned functions and responsibilities that are necessary to pass each clinical rotation. These rotations take place in different various work environments, such as public health and community agencies, homes, schools, clinics, hospitals, and nursing homes. General responsibilities and assigned functions may include assessing a patient, planning and delivering care, performing acute care interventions, providing direct care safely, teaching patients and their family members, and teaching community residents about health and illness. Students must also be competent in reviewing the patient's medical condition, summarizing the patient's chart, assessing health and illness, carrying out the physician's orders, and communicate with all parties. These are basic competencies for students in clinical settings.

To evaluate a student's performance, a certain number of days and a set number of hours are for the clinical instructor's review. Even then, clinical instructors often find that the clinical rotation time is too short. Therefore, *instructors frown on student absences or tardine*ss, as it further minimizes the time available for student evaluation, and are responsible for enforcing all policies pertaining to this conduct.

ABSENCES

This is not to say that clinical educators want students who are ill to care for patients. But *the student is responsible for in-*

forming the instructor the night before or on the day of the clinical experience of an illness.

For a prolonged and unexpected student absence, the routine procedure is for the assigned faculty to discuss the situation and designate a plan of action for that student. Each case needs individual attention by the designated faculty. Clinical instructors are never alone in making these decisions.

Make-Up Assignments

For minor illnesses, a "make-up assignment" or "make-up clinical time" is the routine plan. Some nursing programs allow the student to make up the clinical experience on another day either with the regular clinical instructor or another instructor. Students are required to pay "out of pocket" for this make-up extra time (based on a set fee structure). Other programs routinely prefer to provide "make-up work" for the student. Examples of such work can be a research article critique, a literature review presentation, or the completion of several case studies from a workbook. Make-up work should be collected within a week of the absence. It is wise to check with the program's set coordinator for other examples of acceptable make-up work. Moreover, each nursing program usually has a designated lab area designed for self–directed student learning. Other worthwhile assignments may be extracted from this environment.

Instructors should designate make-up work that can assist the students in meeting the required clinical objectives. However, *constant or prolonged absences are a detriment to the student's overall progress* and prevent successful achievement of the objectives. This leads to a poor clinical grade and clinical/academic failure. *Make sure you track student absences.* It is recommended that at the second absence, the instructor contact the program's level coordinator for feedback on managing this issue. The program may already have a procedure in place for handling this issue.

If you need to devise make-up work, it is wise to have students complete assignments related to the clinical practicum or related to the nursing theory course in which they are currently enrolled. Exhibits 16.1 and 16.2 offer examples of make-up work assignments that you can apply for your student groups.

EXHIBIT 16.1   Written Make-Up Assignments for Clinical Absence

---

A. The instructor will assign a literature review on a medical surgical nursing topic. The paper will be graded on content and the format required for a literature review.

The literature review will include a title page and a reference page (current). It will be a minimum of six pages, with the format and margins as required by the 5th edition of the APA guidelines.

Due date: 10 days from absence.

B. The instructor will assign three case studies to be completed by the following Thursday.

**EXHIBIT 16.2   Oral Make-Up Assignment
for Clinical Absence**

Guidelines for an Ethical–Legal Presentation

1. Select an ethical or legal topic from the pediatric or medical surgical nursing specialties as the basis for a discussion or debate.

2. Review the literature and provide a five-minute presentation (include a written outline to be shared with group) using one of the following techniques:

   - Focus on a recent debate issue.
   - Highlight a recent "news" item on the issue.
   - Present the research problem and identify a question.
   - Present a case study from your experience.
   - Summarize the literature.

3. Lead a five-minute discussion on this topic

4. Bonus points: any creativity brought to the presentation.

TARDINESS

As with absences, the *clinical instructor should monitor student tardiness from the first day* of the clinical experience. Students can be tardy for numerous reasons, such as car problems and road conditions. However, the student should not offer these excuses to explain a pattern of tardiness. If a student arrives late every Tuesday morning, then the student has a responsibility problem and should be evaluated accordingly.

Each time a student is tardy, the instructor should be informed as early as possible. As soon as the student arrives, he or she must immediately seek the clinical instructor for a briefing on what was missed. The clinical instructor can usually assign a late student to work with another student or staff member. Such adjustments depend on the location of the clinical experience, as student responsibilities and duties vary by setting. If a student has a pattern of lateness, that student will probably not meet some of the clinical objectives. This will affect their overall clinical grade. It is recommended that clinical instructors inform the faculty level coordinator to discuss any absent or tardy student—as soon as they can!

Fast facts in a nutshell

- Nursing program instructors value punctuality.
- Clinical absences require make-up work.
- Nursing programs have policies regarding absences and tardiness.

Chapter 17

Unsafe Practice

INTRODUCTION

Standards of care for nursing professionals emphasize safe and competent practice. As a result, most programs have clearly defined policies regarding safe and unsafe practice. There is zero tolerance for any unsafe practice.

In this chapter, you will learn:

1. A detailed example of an unsafe practice event
2. The requirements for the instructor who encounters a similar event.

SAFE PRACTICE

Nursing programs have a moral and ethical responsibility to prepare graduates who will be competent and safe caregivers. This obligation is clearly spelled out by the American Nurses Association (ANA). In some programs, safe practice is documented as adequate knowledge of the nursing process and safe performance of skills, such as patient assessment and medication administration. In other programs, safe practice involves behaviors that uphold the ANA Code of Ethics. Clinical educators must be aware that **the concept of "safe or unsafe practice" is not commonly defined by all nursing programs.** The clinical instructor is encouraged to seek this definition (if applicable) in the student handbook or ask the level coordinator or a faculty contact person if there is a policy and definition.

ANA Code

The ANA's Code of Ethics (2001) requires that "the nurse acts to safeguard the client and public when healthcare and safety are affected by the incompetent, unethical, or illegal practice of any person." Both students and faculty have this ethical duty. As a result, the clinical instructor must strictly uphold this code of ethics in the practicum experience. **Students should be well aware of the rules and standards** before beginning each rotation.

What Is an Unsafe Event?

As discussed earlier, it is incumbent on clinical educators to understand all policies and procedures for evaluating students. Exhibit 17.1 is an example of an unsafe event involving student MaryPat and a clinical instructor. For some, it may be surprising that this is classified as an unsafe event, as it did not cause direct "harm" nor was it classified as a "med error." These are the most commonly thought of unsafe practice events.

However, in this example, the student not only acted beyond her authorized role, she did not follow the nursing process by completing a patient assessment before any intervention. The clinical instructor met with the student the next day and had the student read the written report of the day's event. The student understood she was being cited for unsafe practice and that she had not properly followed the nursing process. The student confirmed her understanding by signing the bottom of the event report sheet.

EXHIBIT 17.1A   Unsafe Practice Event

Clinical instructor, Cindy, was at the opposite end of the hall when she saw her student, MaryPat, looking quite stressed. The clinical instructor quickly made her way into the room of Mary Pat's patient. She observed Mary Pat's apprehensiveness and the fact that the patient's intravenous (IV) bag was empty. Mary Pat's patient had been bathed and was reading the paper on a chair next to her bed. Everything looked neatly organized, but there was a ringing noise coming from the IV pump. It seemed that the IV bag and IV line were empty. Cindy quickly turned off the IV pump, while also clamping the IV bag. Cindy also observed that the IV tubing was looped incorrectly into the IV pump, as a key filter was not attached. She asked Mary-Pat how long the IV had been ringing, and MaryPat answered, "only a few minutes." MaryPat shared that the patient asked to be bathed and then helped into her chair. Cindy informed MaryPat that the pump was ringing because the bag and tubing had air in them. She also added, "Did someone come in and disconnect the tubing from

(continued)

the pump?" MaryPat acknowledged that she had to disconnect the bag and tubing so that she could change the gown after the bath. Cindy picked up the nurse's assessment flow sheet and asked Mary-Pat to join her in the hallway. Once in the hallway she guided MaryPat into the clean utility room, "Do you know what was running in the IV bag?" MaryPat looked hesitant and did not quickly offer an answer but started looking for her handwritten notes from that morning's report. She stood and answered, "Normal saline with potassium?" Cindy turned to MaryPat and commented, "That bag has been infusing with heparin, which you did not document on the morning report. Two weeks ago, you also had a patient with a heparin infusion. We assessed and documented that case together. More important, the tubing was not attached to the pump correctly, so this patient may have received more heparin than she should have. Do you understand that this is a major event? We will have to report this to the primary nurse and the physician. We will also have to fill out an event report and follow the policy accordingly. But, first, let us find the primary nurse to see what he wants us to do next."

That afternoon, after the postconference, Cindy told MaryPat to meet her in her office the next day to discuss the seriousness of the morning's event. She told MaryPat that she saw the event as an "unsafe practice" and would need to share a written report on the situation and follow the policy on unsafe practice as documented in the student handbook. She asked MaryPat if she had any questions regarding her comments. MaryPat said "no," but then she quickly added, " I had taken the IV lines off the pump before . . . when I worked as a patient care technician. I sometimes had to get patients ready for their tests so I detached them from the pumps. The staff nurses have seen me do this many times."

The instructor explained to MaryPat that even though she had worked with IVs as a patient care technician, she was functioning now only as a student—and not as a technician. Therefore, she was not allowed to disconnect IV lines during her clinical rotation without the supervision of the clinical instructor. The clinical instructor also stressed that the role of the student was discussed extensively on orientation day and she also showed MaryPat that it was explicitly stated in writing on the clinical handouts the students received.

The clinical instructor then followed the policy at this particular nursing program by discussing the incident with the level coordinator. At faculty meetings, unsafe practice events are discussed. This raises faculty awareness and draws attention to students who have "patterns" of unsafe practice events in their records. All instructors should have a thorough understanding of the nursing program's policy on unsafe practice (if any). There should not be any ambiguity in the clinical setting regarding the clinical instructor's role in the event of such situations.

ASSESSING SAFE PRACTICE

Because the **primary goal of nursing education is to train safe and competent nurses** who are accountable for their actions, clinical educators have a legal, ethical, and professional responsibility to assess students for safe practice (Smith, McKoy & Richardson, 2001). In some cases, clinical educators may be reluctant to enforce this unsafe practice policy because of unclear direction by their nursing programs. They simply may not have had previous experience in enforcing enforce this policy, or they may not be sure that their student evaluation will be upheld and supported by program officials.

Failing a Student for Unsafe Practice

In addition, **instructors may face challenges from failing students**. Students will usually challenge upsetting academic decisions in a process that some colleges and universities call "grievance." The student's family may also become involved. All of these psychosocial aspects are challenging to the clinical instructor. It is generally more work and aggravation to fail a clinical student than to simply let them pass. However the ethical and legal responsibilities remain. Clinical educators are hired to assess and assist their students. Nursing programs are designed to produce students who can satisfactorily and safely perform skills.

Examples of Unsafe Practice

Instructors should be alerted to examples of unsafe practice events. Additional unsafe events include:

1. The **student has not prepared for assigned tasks.** The student was given an assignment to review all aspects of patient medications before administering them, but he arrives at the clinical day without having looked up or prepared any of the medications.
2. A **student has not reported abnormal vital signs** to the staff nurse or clinical instructor. An adult patient had a temperature of 102 degrees in a postprocedure setting, but the student did not report this event.
3. A **student has given medications without the presence of the clinical instructor.** Students must be made aware that

they are practice nursing under the license and guidance of the clinical instructor. This information is in the rules and guidelines they receive on orientation day. Not following these rules should mandate an unsafe practice report.

Fast facts in a nutshell

- The clinical instructor must be aware of the ANA Code of Ethics
- Each nursing program has its own definition of safe and unsafe practices.

Chapter 18

What Your Students Will Expect of You

INTRODUCTION

Now that you are prepared to enter the world of a clinical nursing instructor, it will be important to focus on what your students will expect of you. You have clearly informed them, on their orientation day, about all of your expectations as well as those of the nursing school. Now it is time to think about their expectations of you.

In this chapter, you will learn:

1. The four important attributes or traits that students expect in a clinical nursing instructor.
2. The ABCs of developing a successful and professional relationship with your students.

STUDENT EXPECTATIONS OF INSTRUCTORS

You have prepared well for your new role as a clinical nursing instructor. You have read this book and used its "blueprints" to prepare for your orientation day, student evaluations, and unit orientation. There is one more lesson to learn.

You know what you expect of yourself, but what do your students expect of you? Although they may never verbalize their expectations, **students require several vital qualities in their instructor.** That is why successful nursing clinical instructors remember to bring their CAPs to clinical each day. The CAP is not the iconic headpiece worn in the past, but rather a pneumonic that captures the essential traits you must always exhibit to your charges:

C   CONSISTENCY
A   APPROACHABILITY
P   PROFICIENCY

CONSISTENCY

Nursing students are usually quite anxious on their first clinical day of each rotation. There often are rumors that upper classmates circulate about the clinical instructor, the unit, and the workload of each rotation. The first day is often marked by shaking legs, nervous stares, and sweaty palms. This is not all bad. It is important for each student to appreciate the seriousness of the responsibility that he or she has at the clinical site, as well as the corresponding burden of responsibility borne by the clinical nursing instructor. In each circumstance, a facility's professional staff is allowing you and your students to enter their domain and care for their clients. The trust that the clients place in the facility is temporarily transferred to you.

The students must realize this and must trust you to help them navigate this unfamiliar territory. They trust you to provide adequate orientation; to establish safe limits and boundaries in terms of their roles; to ask them questions that pinpoint their areas of weakness; and to have a cohesive working relationship with the unit staff that will aid and benefit their education. Students must also be secure in their knowledge of who you are and what you expect. As such, **you must exhibit consistency in your day-to-day oversight** of their activities.

What does this mean? It means that you have to stick to your word and to what you have documented in handouts. If you say that you will e-mail their assignments to them by 4 PM, you must do so. It means that if you say that one journal is due each week and provide the guidelines for it, you stick to that expectation and format. You cannot change the expectations after the rotation begins. Consider the examples in Exhibit 18.1.

EXHIBIT 18.1   Consistency

Case 1

Kate is an instructor with one or two students who complain that the workload of a weekly journal assignment is too much with all of their other course responsibilities. They request that she reduce this assignment. However, most of the other students are having no

(continued)

difficulty completing the task and find the assignment helpful for their learning. Kate changes the assignment to resolve the complaint.

Case 2

Jerry is an instructor who tells his students on orientation day that he requires that they know the category, dose, and side effects of all of their medications. Then, on medication day, he goes further and asks them about chemical composition, actions, and half-life of the meds.

Case Evaluation

In the first case, the instructor lowered her stated expectations, while in the second case, the instructor increased what he originally asked of his students. Both instructors lacked consistency and were ultimately unfair to their students. **Vacillating expectations only serve to undermine student trust** in the instructor.

Trustworthiness

Trustworthiness and consistency are intertwined. To be reliable as a nursing clinical instructor, students should often be able to predict your actions and reactions. For example, if they do not submit their journal to you on the appropriate day, they need to know from the outset that you will subtract 5 points from their grade unless they experienced a real emergency. Everyone, including the star student who is the nursing clinical genius and the struggling student who may be in jeopardy of failure, must know the policy. Consistency demands the same treatment for the same quality of work. **There can be no favoritism.**

Therefore, if you expect the students to be on the unit for clinical at 6:45 AM, then you too are on the unit at that time. While no nursing instructor is immune to the risks of a flat tire, a roadblock, a storm, or other situation that can delay arrival at the clinical site, these situations should be the exceedingly rare exception. Be where you are supposed to be on time.

Evaluation Policies

You also need to **be consistent with your evaluation policies.** If you say that the end of the clinical day is at 1400, do not make an exception for a student who may have an appointment. For example, students will ask to leave early because they have a professional nursing job interview. Keep in mind, however, that clinical time is valuable and already limited, so you do not want to take time away from the experience. In addition, if other students will see you indulge certain exceptions, you will open up Pandora's box, as students will ask for other types of early dismissal requests.

Consistency also means if you tell a student you will supervise her insertion of a urinary Foley catheter in her patient's room in 15 minutes, you are in fact there to supervise her at the appointed time. If an emergency delays you, send a second student down to inform the first student as to why you are not there and make other arrangements. A student will become extremely frustrated if he or she is waiting for your arrival and you do not show. The client loses trust in the student, and the student will lose trust in you.

The trust your students place in you will earned by the fairness and reliability that you consistently project.

APPROACHABILITY

Because students are anxious as they embark on a new clinical rotation, you must establish standards, guidelines, and rules. At the same time, however, **you must remain approachable**. What does this mean? Approachable means that you **explain your rationale and ask for questions**. If there are no questions, you ask students to explain in their own words what they heard you say.

Approachable means that you announce on the first day that you understand that each student is an individual with different learning needs and different experiences. Some of your students may work as aides or nursing technicians in healthcare facilities and have therefore learned many skills of care on the job. Others may have been a care provider in a different kind of facility. You must emphasize that you realize the differences and that all the objectives can be met by each student despite their varying degrees of exposure to working in a healthcare setting. State emphatically that you want students to tell you when they do not know something. The benefits of this policy are shown in Exhibit 18.2.

EXHIBIT 18.2   Approachability

During her psychiatric rotation, a senior student was responsible for taking the blood pressure of the clients on the unit. She seemed very upset by this assignment and explained to the instructor that on her job, she took blood pressure using a noninvasive automatic blood pressure cuff and had therefore forgotten how to take blood pressure manually. It was important for this senior nursing student to feel that the instructor was approachable in this situation. It allowed the instructor to review the student's technique and require her to return to the nursing skills lab for practice.

Fairness

It is vital for students to feel that you are approachable as they deliver care to their clients. If the student makes an error or even thinks that she has made an error, she will be concerned and anxious. At the same time, she should feel that her concern and anxiety are not barriers to immediately coming to you with the problem.

Being approachable does not mean that you are a buddy or friend to your students. It means that they are aware that you are there to help them succeed. Your approachability will be demonstrated by your ability to remain reasonable and emotionally controlled when your assistance is needed concurrently in multiple places, when you are behind in your schedule, or when you are just not feeling up to par. **Remaining approachable is paramount for the safety of the patients and the security of the students caring for them.**

PROFICIENCY

As the instructor, **you are the acknowledged expert**. Your students watch your technique carefully and rely on your advice. The nursing staff depends on your expertise to ensure that no harm comes to patients as a result of student inexperience. So what exactly is your level of expertise in a field whose breadth of information and practice seemingly evolves by the day? Unless you make a continued effort to keep your knowledge current, you cannot discharge your role effectively. See Exhibit 18.3 for an example of the importance of proficiency.

EXHIBIT 18.3   Proficiency

At the start of the Fall semester, Rhonda brought her new class to the med/surg floor on which she had not worked for the past four years. The first day quickly turned into a nightmare, as Rhonda realized that the process of dispensing medications had become automated with optically scanned barcodes. Because of the security embedded in the new technology, she had no means of accessing the system and no idea how to use it once it was accessed. The students were not able to complete the fundamental chore of administering medications, and Rhonda's credibility suffered in the eyes of staff and students alike.

Case Evaluation

How can such an unfortunate situation be avoided? Start by subscribing to professional publications. These timely periodicals can offer valuable information on how research and technical innovation are affecting nursing care, often before these innovations are widely introduced into practice. It is also a good idea to **keep in touch with the nurse manager**, who can be a considerable asset in this regard. Innovations are usually introduced with sufficient lead time to allow for their incorporation into the daily routine. Just as the staff nurses get on-site training, so too should you. Since it may not be appropriate or feasible to participate in the training provided to the nursing staff, take the initiative to **shadow a staff nurse for the day** (with permission of course). This investment of time will pay dividends later, when all student eyes turn to you for instruction in a new skill.

Remember that you too were once a nursing student. The expectations you had of your instructors are likely no different that those that your students now have of you. They depend on you, and they need to trust you. You will earn their trust through consistency, approachability, and proficiency. Among your students you may very well have a future nursing instructor who will emulate the example you set today.

Fast facts in a nutshell

- Your students have many expectations of you.
- Anticipate student expectations and strive to meet them.
- When you enter the clinical site, do not forget your CAP
- Consistency, Approachability, and Proficiency.

Chapter 19

Conclusion

INTRODUCTION

The major purpose of this book was to provide specific and practical information and guidelines for clinical nursing instructors. Many of these instructors work hard to perform a role whose complexities and frustrations are often under-recognized. A clinical instructor has one of the most challenging and potentially rewarding positions in the nursing profession. Today, more than ever, it is a role that every state needs to fill in a multitude of programs.

In this chapter, you will learn:

1. To summarize each chapter in this book.
2. How the authors intended this book to be used.

PURPOSE AND ORGANIZATION OF THIS BOOK

This book has seven major sections and 18 chapters. The chapters provided elemental information applicable to all clinical nursing instructors. Some offered knowledge about the mechanics of clinical instruction, while others assisted a new instructor in organizing his or her work. However, this book does not provide all the information necessary to teach student nurses. It is not intended to replace the much needed graduate programs that focus on teaching registered nurses how to become effective clinical educators. **Advanced education focused on the teaching role is highly necessary.**

This book is really intended to assist those who have transitioned from the practice role to that of educator. It can serve as **a supplemental guide or handbook for those who want to refresh their knowledge** about the clinical instructor role.

Parts and Chapters

Part I, which includes Chapters 1 and 2, is an **introduction to the clinical instructor role.** The first presents the basic facts of clinical teaching and includes the expectations of many novice instructors. You are also asked to assess your knowledge base role. Chapter 2 asks you to assess your knowledge of standard rules and policies in nursing education.

Part II focuses on **the clinical teaching workload.** Chapters 3 reviews the priority tasks for the clinical instructor as he or she works not only with students, but also with staff. Chapter 4 highlights the orientation day and provides a sample template for that day. The orientation day is a key time for communication between the instructor and the students. Chapter 5 discusses the major responsibilities of the clinical instructor's role that will enhance the instructor's relationships with the staff and his or her students.

Part III offers **a strategy for maximizing the limited observation and supervision time** inherent in the clinical rotation world. That is why many instructors attempt to "see it early." Chapters 6 and 7 reviews characteristics of "high fliers" and "not-so-high fliers." High fliers are students who will pass the course and possibly received a higher than average grade. The "not-so-high fliers" are those who may receive lower grades than most or are at risk for course failure.

The key aspects of the clinical evaluation are presented in Part IV. Chapter 8 discusses the importance of student self-evaluation. Students should realize that self-evaluation is a responsibility they will carry into their professional lives as registered nurses. To assist instructors to become more efficient in evaluating students, anecdotal notetaking is highlighted in Chapter 9 as an advantageous strategy. Chapter 10 provides a more elaborate discussion of warning signs for students who are in danger of failing. Unsatisfactory performance behavior is identified in this chapter. Chapter 11 presents the most common grading systems used in nursing programs: letter/number and pass/fail, or satisfactory/unsatisfactory, grading systems.

In Part V we referenced **communication as a key element** in most nursing clinical courses. The communication of students is observed in their behavior with patients and in their behavior at group discussion sessions or conferences that take place before and/ or after the clinical day. Chapter 12 discusses preconference elements and chapter 13 focuses on postconferences.

Part VI addresses one of the most difficult challenges faced by the clinical instructor—the **assignment of patients to each student.** Dealing with unplanned events and their effects on the student-patient assignment is highlighted in Chapter 14. The chapter also provides an overview of alternative assignments to optimize the clinical experience of students in any setting.

The last section, Part VII, focuses on **essential competencies found in most programs.** Chapter 16 discusses absences and tardiness policies as it applies to the student in clinical rotations. Chapter 17 provides a description of unsafe practice as behaviors not consistent with those documented in the ANA's Code of Ethics. Safe practice policies are now common in most nursing programs. Finally, Chapter 18 highlights important tips necessary to have a successful and professional relationship with your students.

Fast Facts in a Nutshell

Each chapter includes "**fast facts in a nutshell,**" a feature that highlights key elements of the chapter. Some chapters also provide questionnaires or exercises for you to complete. These are intended to assist in your understanding of the role of clinical nursing instructor. Finally, the appendix includes several key items that will help you prepare for the role. Items in the appendices are supplemental material for the experienced instructor, however some novice instructors may find them to be more valuable, especially if they have yet to embark on their first clinical instructor assignment.

DYNAMICS OF CLINICAL INSTRUCTION

As you read each chapter, you will realize the respect the authors have for clinical instruction and the academic goal of providing quality-nursing education to future nurses. It is a challenging task to educate a student nurse. We have attempted, in our own way, to provide you—the clinical instructor—with some information about the basic dynamics of clinical instruction. As mentioned earlier, we have years of experience in the role because we truly enjoy it! We commend you for your bravery in embarking on this endeavor.

You should **have fun and be open to humor** in the role. If you are relaxed, this will be conveyed to your students and will enhance their performance. Moreover, you will quickly realize that there are many surprises in the role. Some students will forward you a "thank you" card at the end of the practicum. Also, do not be surprised if they seek you at graduation. They may invite you to the final year student dinner or the pinning ceremony. Student nurses will become indebted to you and will want to visit even after graduation from the program. It is a remarkable reward to have that kind of effect on your students.

Furthermore, remember the need to **"take care" of yourself.** If you are not a good role model to your students for "self-care," that essential lesson will not be learned. Take breaks, eat lunch, sit down, and always tell yourself that you are attempting to accomplish an exciting and ambitious role.

You have taken a very important step in your professional nursing career. The fact that you have read this book shows that you are truly interested in becoming an effective and successful teacher. You have made a commitment to become one of those clinical instructors mentioned in the Foreword by Dr. Slaninka, "as the one who made me the nurse I am today!" **You have made a commitment to be an effective clinical nursing instructor.** Congratulations in joining the club!

Appendix A

Guidelines for
Clinical Orientation Day

WELCOME TO 3 C

Orientation day begins exactly at 8 am sharp. Meet at **the Barden Lobby**. Directions are provided and you also can access the clinical settings Web site at www.lifecare.org.

September 1, 2008
This is a regular clinical day with time allocated for lunch. The schedule is 8 AM to 2 PM.

Bring BP cuff, stethoscope, pen, paper, notebook and wear full uniform with identification badge per student handbook.

Expectations for students will be discussed during this orientation day.

Park in the hospital garage and you will receive parking vouchers for each day. They cannot be replaced. The fee for parking at TMH is $8.00/day without vouchers.

There will be a med quiz on this orientation day per level policy. You must pass this quiz to begin giving meds at the site. Safe knowledge and administration of meds are evaluated at all times.

3 C is an approximately 30-bed surgical unit. There are also designated beds for short-stay after surgical procedures. Please review surgical procedures in your med-surg and Smith textbooks. You will probably have an opportunity to irrigate Nasogastric tubes, change dressings, provide postop care, discharge instructions, give subcutaneous insulin and Lovenox, complete assessments, perform sterile gloving for hygiene and personal care, prioritize care, and review pain management. Go to the Operating room, endoscopy unit, and work with a staff nurse.

Please begin to review all of the above procedures. You are expected to review any skill needed in the lab with Marlene if you have any questions or need to practice. I expect you to have reviewed all of the above skills and have practiced in the lab before a clinical opportunity to perform that skill occurs.

This is a fast-pace unit, and there are registered nurses, patient care techs, and aides, unit secretary.

Unit coordinator is Diane Marag

Unit manager is Mary Beth Brouty.

Unit number on 3 C is 610-626-3635.

I look forward to working with you, and the staff on 3 C are happy to be working with you.

Susan Stabler Haas
Distributed on 8/30/08

Appendix B

Clinical Journal: NSL/NSG 423

WRITTEN ASSIGNMENT: CLINICAL JOURNAL

Instructor: Susan Stabler-Haas

Starting *week 2* of this rotation: Students must submit a clinical journal on at least one of the clients that he or she cared for the previous week. The student must be able to *verbalize* nursing actions and rationale during the clinical day for the patients to whom they are assigned. Examples will be provided. Clinical journals are to be submitted weekly on Tuesday at postconference.

WRITTEN FORMAT OF CLINICAL JOURNAL

INCLUDE YOUR GOALS AND OBJECTIVES FOR THE WEEK IN YOUR CLINICAL JOURNAL

1. PATIENT DATA
   a. Diagnoses
   b. PMH/PSH (past medical and surgical history)

   c. Pathophysiology of diagnoses (cite)
   d. Must compare your client's diagnosis to the textbook
      and cite info from text (cite source)

2. DOCUMENT "SYSTEMS" ASSESSMENT
   a. (See 2nd page)

3. DIAGNOSTIC DATA – LABWORK – NURSING
   IMPLICATIONS
   a. Report *potential* Diagnostics pertinent to diagnoses
      (i.e., chest x-ray results for CHF)
   b. Report any *actual* abnormal lab work and analyze levels
      r/t client.

4. NURSE MANAGEMENT PLAN – Document:
   a. Two priority nursing diagnoses.
   b. One STG per each diagnosis (patient outcome) meas-
      urable.
   c. Two nursing interventions per goal.
   d. Evaluate each intervention.

5. CLIENT EDUCATION
   a. Identify and analyze teaching needs (actual or poten-
      tial) of client.

6. MEDICATIONS
   All medications that the client received during your shift
   must be listed. You must list the name of the medications,
   the indication for the med, lab work needed for this med,
   nursing care, and dosage.

Example: Lovenex: Anticoagulant Prevention of thromboembolism phenomena following surgical procedures, prevention of such disorders when patient on bed rest.

Labs: monitor CBC, platelet count check for black tarry stools, hematuria, fall in blood pressure, signs of bleeding.

Nursing: check for signs of bleeding, gums, stool, urine. Check for bruising.

Dosage: sc (adults) 30 mg. Twice daily start within 24 hours of surgery.

Antidote: Protamine Sulfate.

Reason this patient received med. Patient had surgery and was immobilized, prophylactic.

7. How you feel about the week and your experience.

8. SELF-EVALUATION AND REFLECTION
   (Minimum of 2 paragraphs)

   Reflect on your week: (A) pertinent feelings, and thoughts about the nursing role. (B) Critique your performance as a student nurse. (C) Did you achieve your goals? (D) What would you do differently? ** Write as if you were documenting in a log or diary.

EVALUATION METHOD: CLINICAL JOURNALS will be evaluated based on the evaluative statements from the Clinical Evaluation Tool.

9. **Evaluate** the client's psychological health. Ask the two following questions:
   a. Have you experienced the feeling of sadness over the last two weeks?
   b. Have you lost interest in activities or things that you usually enjoy doing?

Document your assessment of the client's mental state.

Appendix C

4 C Clinical Assignment Sheet

STUDENT	ROOM NUMBER	PATIENT DATA
Claire	Day with nurse	Rose or Jan
Kristen	63 **Meds**	This was Claire's pt. last week. Resp. failure, post MI, post filter inf. Vena cava, Isolation (contact) c.Diff?? Meds: Heparin sub-q, Heparin I.V in PICC line, protonix ivpb, lactinex, vancomycin, vasotec, lanoxin, coreg, novolog flexpen
Cara	53 54	Pancreatitis, c. diff May have companion with her. Did not get diagnosis

(continued)

STUDENT	ROOM NUMBER	PATIENT DATA
Claire	Day with nurse	Rose or Jan
Neil	**Meds** 58	Pneumonia, hyponatremia, pulmonary hypertension Meds: albuterol inhalation, protonix, senokot, solu-medrol IV (20mg.), cardizem cd, colace, lanoxin, humbid LA, A.S.A, tylenol
Karen	O.R	
Amy	59 **MEDS**	Recurrent pneumonia, tube feeding via peg, dsg. Change, Meds: heparin sub-q, heparin IV via PICC, folic acid, ducalox supp., novolin R innolet, albuterol inhalant, MSO4 IV, lorazepan IV
Katie	69	Diabetic ketoacidosis, Blood sugar of 1100 on 10/30. Picc, MRSA,
Casandra	Endo	,.
Beth	79 **MEDS**	This was Casandra's client last week. Contact isolation. PICC flushed, nystatin cream, lopressor, lasix 40 IVP, lac-hytrin 12% topical, alprazolam, albuterol/ipratropium,

References

American Nurses Association (2001). *Code of ethics for nurses with interpretive statements.* Retrieved March 21, 2008 from http://nursingworld.org/ethics/code/protected_nwcoe813.htm

American Association of Colleges of Nursing (1999). *AACN position statement. Nursing education's agenda for the 21st century.* Washington, DC: Author.

Gaberson, K.B. & Oermann, M. H. (1999). *Evaluation and teaching in nursing education.* New York: Springer Publishing Company.

Potter, P., & Perry, A. (2005). *Fundamentals of Nursing.* St. Louis: Missouri.

Scanlon, J. M, Care,W. D. & Gressler, S. (2001). Dealing with the unsafe student in clinical practice. *Nurse Educator, 26*(1), 23–27.

Smith, M. H. McKoy, Y. D. & Richardson, J. (2001). Legal issues related to dismissing students for clinical deficiencies. *Nurse Educator, 26*(1), 33–38.

Teeter, M. (2001). Formula for success: Addressing unsatisfactory clinical performance. *Nurse Educator, 30*(3), 91–92.

Wink. D. M. (1995). The effective clinical conference. *Nursing Outlook, 43,* 29–32.

Index